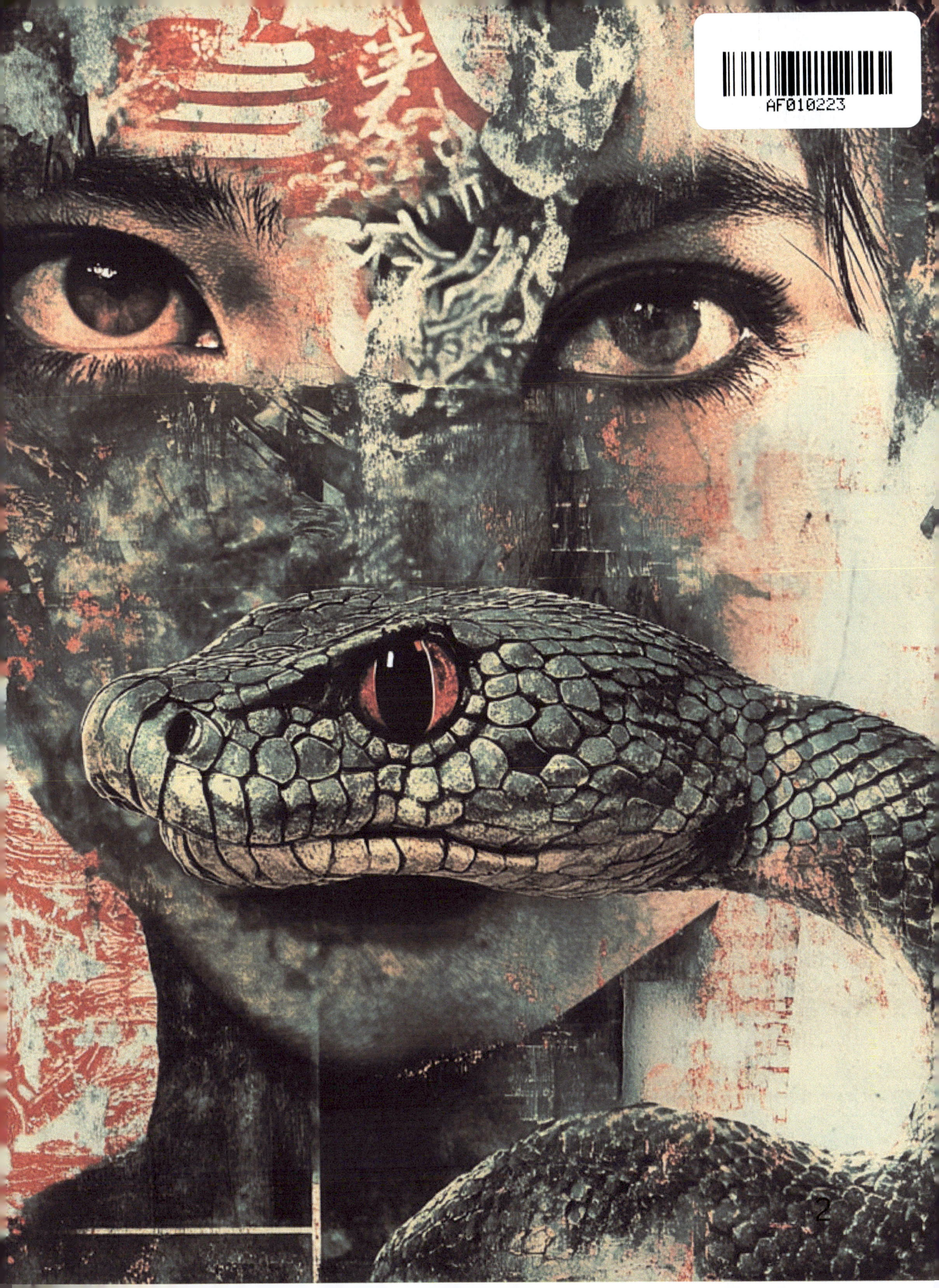

CONTENTS

The Year of the Snake	5
Progress without Pressure	11
AWMA Writing Competition	19
Aikido Love	24
12 Steps for Learning Kata	32
Beat the Heat this Summer	38
Never Too Late...	47
Understanding of Fight or Flight	54
An Equation for Excellence	63
Raising the Bar in Coaching	64
The Enduring Legacy of Jan de Jong	68
Open a Dojo	74
Pin'an Kata	80
The Origins & Evolution of Coloured Belts	84
Recipes from Marty's Kitchen	88
From Couch to Karate	92
IMBA	96
Dojo Doctor	99

Dear Readers,

As we welcome 2025 and the Year of the Snake, I'm reminded of what martial arts teaches us about renewal and adaptation. Just as the snake sheds its skin, we too must sometimes shed old habits to grow.

This issue brings together stories of transformation. We will learn about one practitioner's courageous return to karate after decades away – a testament that it's never too late to begin again. In Leanne Canning's Progress Without the Pressure, we explore how steady, mindful practice often yields better results than rushing toward arbitrary goals.

I'm particularly excited to announce our partnership with the Albury Wodonga Martial Arts (AWMA). The club is running a writing competition as part of their 10th anniversary celebration. Martial artists from around the country are welcome to enter with all proceeds benefitting YES Unlimited. I'm honoured to serve as a judge and we are very proud to be showcasing the winning entries later this year.

Attila Halasz returns with Aikido Love to remind us that martial arts can transform not just our bodies, but our hearts. Sometimes the most meaningful discoveries happen when we least expect them. I am looking forward to his next instalment.

Whether you're setting new goals, returning to training, or deepening your current practice, remember that every journey has its own pace. As we enter the Year of the Snake, let's embrace its qualities of patience, wisdom, and graceful movement.

Yours sincerely,
Vanessa McKay

COPYRIGHT

All content published in MAMA (Marital Arts Magazine Australia), including articles, images, and other media, is the property of the magazine and is protected by copyright law. The author retains the copyright to their individual work, but by submitting their work to MAMA, they grant the magazine an exclusive, perpetual, and irrevocable license to publish and distribute their work in all formats, including print, digital, and online media. No part of MAMA may be reproduced, distributed, or transmitted in any form or by any means, including photocopying, recording, or other electronic or mechanical methods, without the prior written permission of the magazine.

MAMA respects the intellectual property rights of others and expects its contributors and readers to do the same. If you believe that your copyrighted work has been used in a way that constitutes copyright infringement, please contact MAMA immediately. Additionally, any use of MAMA trademarks, including the magazine's name and logo, without prior written authorization from the magazine, is prohibited.

MAMA strives to showcase original and unique content, and as such, does not accept any submissions that have been previously published or that are under consideration by other publications. By submitting their work to MAWA Magazine, the author confirms that their work is original and has not been published or submitted elsewhere.

In addition, MAMA reserves the right to edit all submissions for grammar, style, and clarity, and to reject any submission that does not adhere to the magazine's standards or guidelines. The magazine also reserves the right to remove or modify any content that is deemed inappropriate or offensive, at its sole discretion.

MAMA acknowledges and respects the rights of all individuals and groups and will not publish any content that promotes hate speech, discrimination, or any form of violence. The magazine also respects the privacy of its contributors and readers and will not share or sell any personal information to third parties without prior written consent.

By submitting their work to MAMA, the author agrees to abide by these copyright specifics and to grant the magazine the rights outlined in this statement. The author also certifies that their work is original and does not infringe on the rights of any third party. MAMA reserves the right to modify these copyright specifics at any time without prior notice.

If you have any questions or concerns regarding these copyright specifics, please contact MAMA at info@martialartsmagazineaustralia.com

The Year of the Wood Snake

DRAGON YEARS
 2024: FEB 10, 2024 JAN 28, 2025
 2012: JAN 23, 2012 FEB 9, 2013
 2000: FEB 5, 2000 JAN 23, 2001
 1988: FEB 17, 1988 FEB 5, 1989
 1976: JAN 31, 1976 FEB 17, 1977
 1964: FEB 13, 1964 FEB 1, 1965

TIGER YEARS:
 2022: FEB 1, 2022 JAN 21, 2023
 2010: FEB 14, 2010 FEB 2, 2011
 1998: JAN 28, 1998 FEB 15, 1999
 1986: FEB 9, 1986 JAN 28, 1987
 1974: JAN 23, 1974 FEB 10, 1975
 1962: FEB 5, 1962 JAN 24, 1963

RAT YEARS:
 2020: JAN 25, 2020 FEB 11, 2021
 2008: FEB 7, 2008 JAN 25, 2009
 1996: FEB 19, 1996 FEB 6, 1997
 1984: FEB 2, 1984 FEB 19, 1985
 1972: JAN 16, 1972 FEB 2, 1973
 1960: JAN 28, 1960 FEB 14, 1961

DOG YEARS:
 2018: FEB 16, 2018 FEB 4, 2019
 2006: JAN 29, 2006 FEB 17, 2007
 1994: FEB 10, 1994 JAN 30, 1995
 1982: JAN 25, 1982 FEB 12, 1983
 1970: FEB 6, 1970 JAN 26, 1971

ROOSTER YEARS:
 2017: JAN 28, 2017 FEB 15, 2018
 2005: FEB 9, 2005 JAN 28, 2006
 1993: JAN 23, 1993 FEB 9, 1994
 1981: FEB 5, 1981 JAN 24, 1982
 1969: FEB 17, 1969 FEB 5, 1970

HORSE YEARS:
 2014: JAN 31, 2014 FEB 18, 2015
 2002: FEB 12, 2002 JAN 31, 2003
 1990: JAN 27, 1990 FEB 14, 1991
 1978: FEB 7, 1978 JAN 27, 1979
 1966: JAN 21, 1966 FEB 8, 1967

RABBIT YEARS:
 2023: JAN 22, 2023 FEB 9, 2024
 2011: FEB 3, 2011 JAN 22, 2012
 1999: FEB 16, 1999 FEB 4, 2000
 1987: JAN 29, 1987 FEB 16, 1988
 1975: FEB 11, 1975 JAN 30, 1976
 1963: JAN 25, 1963 FEB 12, 1964

OX YEARS:
 2021: FEB 12, 2021 JAN 31, 2022
 2009: JAN 26, 2009 FEB 13, 2010
 1997: FEB 7, 1997 JAN 27, 1998
 1985: FEB 20, 1985 FEB 8, 1986
 1973: FEB 3, 1973 JAN 22, 1974
 1961: FEB 15, 1961 FEB 4, 1962

PIG YEARS:
 2019: FEB 5, 2019 JAN 24, 2020
 2007: FEB 18, 2007 FEB 6, 2008
 1995: JAN 31, 1995 FEB 18, 1996
 1983: FEB 13, 1983 FEB 1, 1984
 1971: JAN 27, 1971 JAN 15, 1972

GOAT/SHEEP YEARS:
 2015: FEB 19, 2015 FEB 7, 2016
 2003: FEB 1, 2003 JAN 21, 2004
 1991: FEB 15, 1991 FEB 3, 1992
 1979: JAN 28, 1979 FEB 15, 1980
 1967: FEB 9, 1967 JAN 29, 1968

MONKEY YEARS:
 2016: FEB 8, 2016 JAN 27, 2017
 2004: JAN 22, 2004 FEB 8, 2005
 1992: FEB 4, 1992 JAN 22, 1993
 1980: FEB 16, 1980 FEB 4, 1981
 1968: JAN 30, 1968 FEB 16, 1969

SNAKE YEARS:
 2013: FEB 10, 2013 JAN 30, 2014
 2001: JAN 24, 2001 FEB 11, 2002
 1989: FEB 6, 1989 JAN 26, 1990
 1977: FEB 18, 1977 FEB 6, 1978
 1965: FEB 2, 1965 JAN 20, 1966

The Snake year brings a unique combination of the Snake's wisdom and intuition with the Wood element's growth and flexibility. Wood energy promotes new beginnings, growth, and expansion, while the Snake represents intelligence, grace, and transformation.

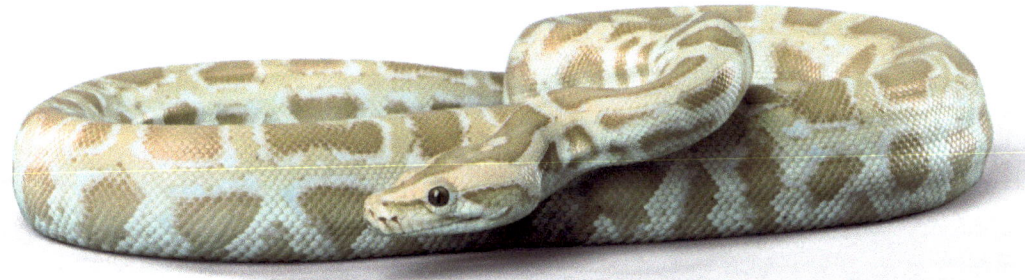

Rat

General Outlook: A year of unexpected opportunities and intellectual growth.

Strengths: Your water element nourishes the year's wood energy, creating favorable conditions

Challenges: Need to avoid overthinking and hesitation.

Prosperity Tips: Focus on educational pursuits and skill development. Build strategic partnerships in the first half of the year. Invest in long term projects starting in spring. Keep written records of your ideas and inspiration.

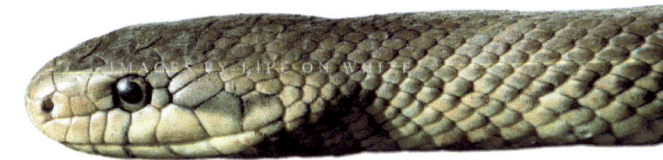

Ox

General Outlook: A year requiring adaptation and flexibility.
Strengths: Your steady nature helps navigate changes.

Challenges: Earth element may feel destabilized by wood energy.

Prosperity Tips: Embrace change rather than resist it.
Focus on personal development and learning new skills.
Build strong support networks.
Practice mindfulness and stress management.

Tiger

General Outlook: Highly favorable year with natural alignment.

Strengths: Your wood nature resonates perfectly with the year's energy.

Challenges: Avoid overconfidence

Prosperity Tips: Take bold initiatives, especially in career. Invest in personal brand-ing. Balance ambition with prac-tical planning.

Rabbit

General Outlook: A year of continued growth and refine-ment.

Strengths: Natural wood energy amplified by the year.

Challenges: Risk of spreading yourself too thin.

Prosperity Tips: Focus on quality over quantity in projects. Nurture existing relationships. Invest in health and wellness. Create detailed action plans for goals.

Dragon

General Outlook: Transition year requiring strategic thinking.

Strengths: Natural leadership qualities enhanced.

Challenges: Earth energy may feel unsettled.

Prosperity Tips: Build on the previous year's momen-tum. Focus on consoli-dation rather than expan-sion. Strengthen family bonds. Invest in property or long term assets.

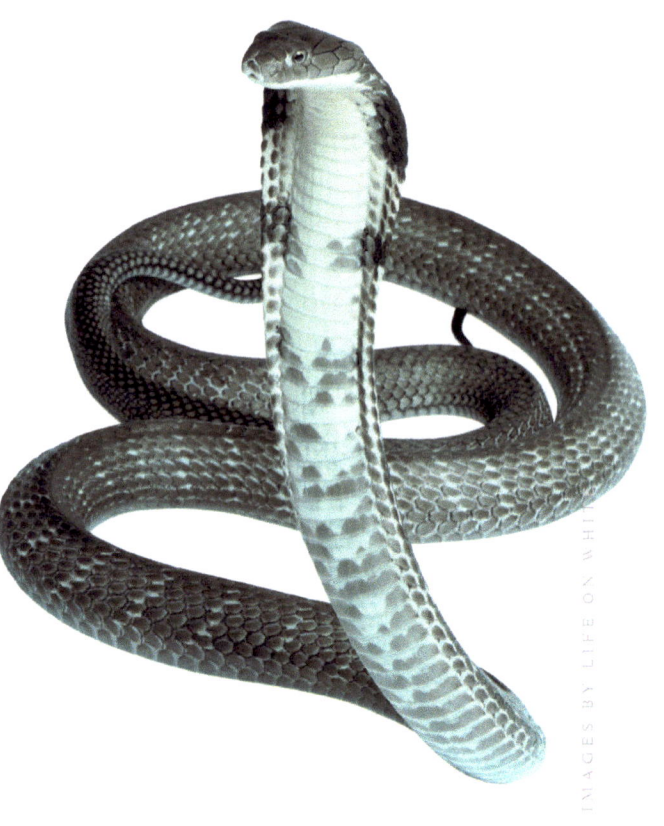

Snake

General Outlook: Your year of personal power and transformation.

Strengths: Enhanced intuition and personal magnetism.

Challenges: Balancing personal needs with obligations.

Prosperity Tips: Take calculated risks in career. Trust your intuition in important decisions. Focus on self-improvement. Develop new income streams.

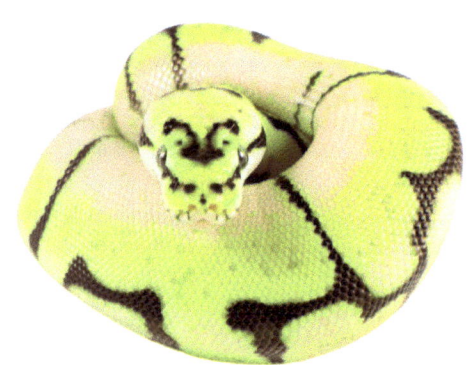

Horse

General Outlook: Dynamic year with significant potential.

Strengths: Fire energy boosted by wood element.

Challenges: Managing impulsiveness.

Prosperity Tips: Channel energy into creative projects. Build professional partnerships. Invest in education and skills. Practice patience in decision making.

Goat

General Outlook: Year of personal growth through challenge.

Strengths: Adaptability in changing circumstances.

Challenges: Earth energy feeling unsettled.

Prosperity Tips: Focus on building stable foundations. Invest in self-care and wellness. Strengthen existing partnerships. Develop multiple income sources.

Monkey

General Outlook: Year requiring strategic adaptation.

Strengths: Natural cleverness helps navigate challenges.

Challenges: Metal element conflicts with wood energy.

Prosperity Tips: Make your focus innovation and creativity. Build strategic alliances. Invest in technology and learning. Maintain flexibility in plans.

Rooster

General Outlook: Year of personal reinvention.

Strengths: Ability to spot opportunities in change.

Challenges: Metal element faces wood's pressure

Prosperity Tips: Focus on personal branding. Develop new skills and competencies. Build strong professional networks. Maintain financial conservatism.

Dog

General Outlook: Year of social opportunity and growth.

Strengths: Loyalty and reliability appreciated.

Challenges: Earth energy requires grounding.

Prosperity Tips: Focus on relationship building. Invest in community connections. Develop leadership skills. Practice consistent saving habits.

Pig

General Outlook: Highly favorable year for growth.

Strengths: Water element nurtures wood energy.

Challenges: Avoid overindulgence.

Prosperity Tips: Focus on personal development. Invest in education and skills. Build long-term investments. Maintain work life balance.

General Prosperity Tips for all Signs in 2025

1. Embrace Growth Mindset
   The Wood element encourages learning and development
   Stay open to new opportunities and changes
   Invest in education and skill development

2. Practice Strategic Thinking
   Snake energy promotes wisdom and careful planning
   Take time to analyze situations before acting
   Consider long term implications of decisions

3. Build Relationships
   Wood element supports relationship growth
   Network actively but authentically
   Strengthen existing connections

4. Financial Management
   Diversify investments
   Create multiple income streams
   Save consistently
   Plan for long term security

5. Health and Wellness
   Balance work and rest
   Practice stress management
   Maintain regular exercise
   Focus on preventive health measures

Remember: Chinese astrology is meant to guide and inspire rather than dictate. Use these insights as a framework for personal growth while maintaining your own judgment and wisdom in decision making.

Progress Without the Pressure
By Leanne Canning at Women Aware Defence

Why is it we're often our worst critics, even in the dojo? Martial artists put insane amounts of pressure on themselves—trying to perfect every movement, every kata, every sparring session. But here's the truth: no one, not even the black-belt grandmasters, gets it all right every time. And that's okay. Being too hard on yourself doesn't make you better; it just makes training less enjoyable.

LET'S TALK ABOUT WHY IT'S TIME TO EASE UP AND STILL GROW STRONGER, BOTH ON AND OFF THE MAT.

Self-Criticism
We all have that little voice inside our heads, pushing us to do better or calling us out on mistakes. For martial artists, this critical voice often goes into overdrive. While a bit of self-correction can help improve skills, too much can crush our confidence and progress. Let's break down what drives this self-criticism and how it impacts training.

WHY DO SO MANY OF US FEEL LIKE WE'RE NOT GOOD ENOUGH ON THE MATS?

Roots of Self-Criticism

Here are some common reasons martial artists may struggle with self-criticism:

Perfectionism: Martial arts demand precision. When we don't land that perfect kick or stance, it's tempting to be our harshest judge.

Comparison to Others: Watching a teammate move flawlessly or gain a promotion can trigger self-comparisons, leaving us feeling inadequate.

Martial Arts as Identity: If being a martial artist is a core part of who you are, any mistake can feel like a personal failure.

Past Experiences: Maybe a coach or instructor's feedback stuck with you a little too much. That harsh tone can replay in your head like a bad movie.

Ever catch yourself replaying a failed sparring session in your mind? That's self-criticism feeding off these roots. Recognising where it comes from is the first step toward shutting it down.

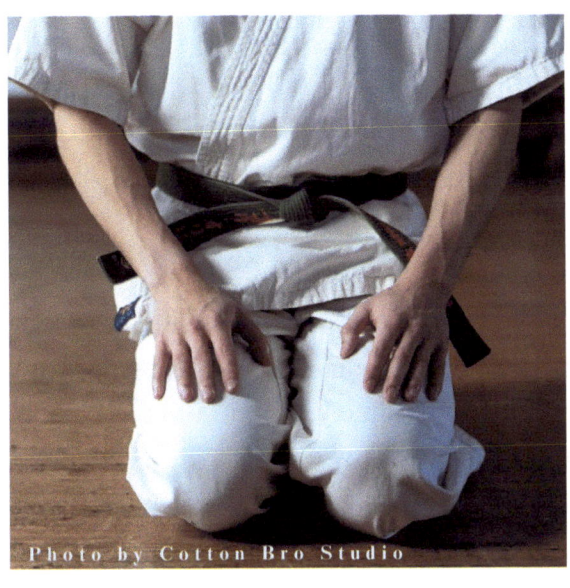

Impact on Training and Performance

ONCE SELF-CRITICISM SNEAKS INTO YOUR MIND, IT CAN AFFECT YOUR ENTIRE TRAINING EXPERIENCE.

Decreased Confidence: Harping on your mistakes makes you doubt yourself, holding back progress.

Hindered Performance: Thinking about failure during sparring or drills means you're not focusing on the present, slowing down reaction times.

Burnout Risk: Constant self-blame can suck the joy out of training, making it feel like a chore rather than a passion.

Fear of Failure: When mistakes seem catastrophic, you might avoid taking risks or trying new techniques altogether.

Martial arts isn't about being perfect. It's about improvement. Letting self-criticism dominate can rob you of that growth. The next time it kicks in, remind yourself: mistakes are just stepping stones to success.

A Positive Mindset

Every martial artist knows the mental battles are just as intense as the physical ones. Whether you're perfecting techniques or recovering from setbacks, a positive mindset is essential for growth. It's not just about getting things right; it's about how you respond when they go wrong. Let's dive into actionable ways to shift from being too critical to approaching training—and life—with kindness.

Celebrate Small Wins

As martial artists, we often measure success in big moments—tournaments, belt promotions, or mastering challenging techniques. But here's a question: why skip over the little victories? Whether it's nailing a single punch in a combination or finally getting low enough in a horse stance, your progress is made up of these small moments.

Celebrate your progress:

Take a mental note when a drill feels smoother than last week.

Share your improvements with training partners—they'll cheer you on!

Reward yourself (hello, favourite snack?) after tough, focused sessions.

Small wins stack like bricks, building the foundation of your confidence. Each one deserves recognition, no matter how tiny it might seem.

Practice Self-Compassion

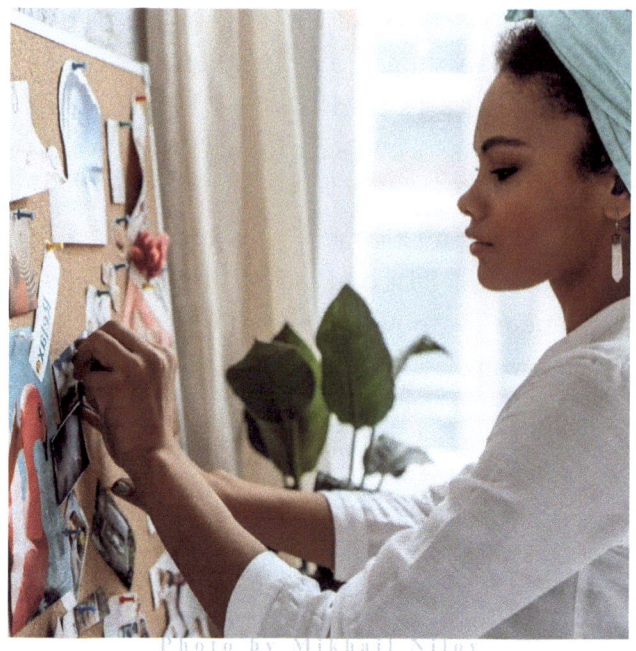
Photo by Mikhail Nilov

Think about how you'd respond to a struggling beginner who's frustrated because they can't land a kick. You wouldn't criticise them, right? You'd want to encourage and guide them. So why not be the same way toward yourself?

Practicing self-compassion means letting go of the need to be perfect 24/7. It's okay to not get every move right. Growth comes from effort, not flawlessness. Replace negative thoughts like "I'll never get this" with simple affirmations:

"I'VE DONE HARD THINGS BEFORE. I CAN DO THIS TOO."

"MISTAKES MEAN I'M LEARNING."

Remember, imperfection isn't weakness—it's human. The dojo isn't a courtroom; we don't need to pass judgment on every misstep. By treating ourselves with kindness, we create space for improvement without unnecessary pressure.

Visualisation Techniques

Visualisation isn't just for athletes at the top of their game; it's for all of us pushing to get better. It's the mental warm-up before the physical motion. Martial artists can use it to slow down those self-critical thoughts and channel energy into achieving their goals—both on and off the mat. Think of it like rehearsing your success in your mind before stepping into action. Let's break it down.

Imagining Success

Picture this: you're about to drill a complex kick combo or grapple with a tougher sparring partner. Instead of spiraling into "What if I mess up?", try visualising yourself executing the move flawlessly. Imagine the snap of your kick, the sound of your foot hitting the pad, and the approving nod of your instructor.

Why does this work? Your brain doesn't completely separate imagined experiences from real ones. When we see ourselves succeeding—even if only in our minds—it builds confidence. It sets the stage for real-world wins by telling your nervous system, "I've got this."

Visualisation also cuts through that inner critic. If you're too busy focusing on success, there's no room left for doubts. So before your next practice, close your eyes for a few quiet moments. Walk through the technique mentally, paying attention to every detail. Then get moving, knowing you already nailed it once in your head.

Setting Realistic Goals

Let's be real: thinking about success is great, but it works best alongside realistic goals.

Unrealistic expectations can gnaw away at anyone, especially martial artists striving for perfection.

When setting goals, it's not about going from white belt to black belt overnight. Break things down:

1. Short-term targets: Start with perfecting a single move, like improving the speed of your roundhouse.

2. Mid-term focus: Think about stringing a combo together under pressure in sparring.

3. Long-term wins: Visualise acing your next belt test. What does it feel like to tie that new belt around your waist?

Smaller, defined goals do more than keep us motivated—they're an antidote to self-criticism. When goals are achievable, failure feels less like a crushing defeat and more like a stepping stone. Consistently check small wins off your list will keep that inner voice happier.

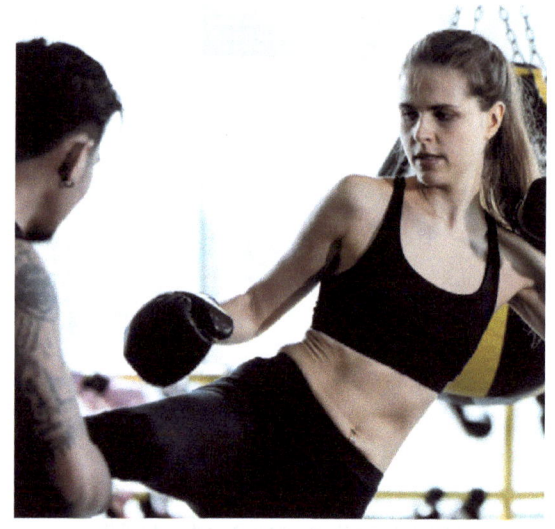

Visualisation is like having a personal highlight reel at your disposal. With it, you can replay and rehearse success until it feels natural. Paired with smart, realistic goals, it's the perfect technique to shut down self-doubt while taking control of progress. Now go ahead— imagine the version of yourself thriving.

Finding Support in the Martial Arts Community

Training in martial arts can sometimes feel like a solo battle, but it doesn't have to be. One of the incredible things about martial arts is the community it builds. Connecting with others not only boosts your skills but also helps you navigate self-doubt and stay motivated. Let's talk about finding support and why it's a game-changer for anyone who's too hard on themselves.

Mentorship and Guidance

Every martial artist benefits from having someone a little wiser, a little more experienced, to show them the way. Mentors aren't just instructors who teach you how to punch or perform a kata; they're your guides in navigating challenges, both on the mats and in your head.

Think of a mentor as a compass. When you feel lost—frustrated with your progress or stuck on a technique—they point you in the right direction. They've walked the same path you're on, so their advice comes from real experience. Leaning on their wisdom isn't cheating; it's necessary.

What does seeking mentorship look like?

·Ask questions: Don't be shy! Whether it's about technique, mindset, or injury recovery, they're there to help.

·Observe their habits: Watch how they train, how they recover from mistakes, and how they deal with pressure.

Mentors help you see your potential when your inner critic is on overdrive. They've been there before and understand the pressures you're feeling. Having someone cheer for you and guide you builds confidence quicker than going it alone.

Building a Support Network

Martial arts isn't just about what happens on the mats; the relationships built during training make it so much more rewarding. Whether it's sweating through drills together or laughing about sparring mishaps after class, a good training group creates a sense of belonging.

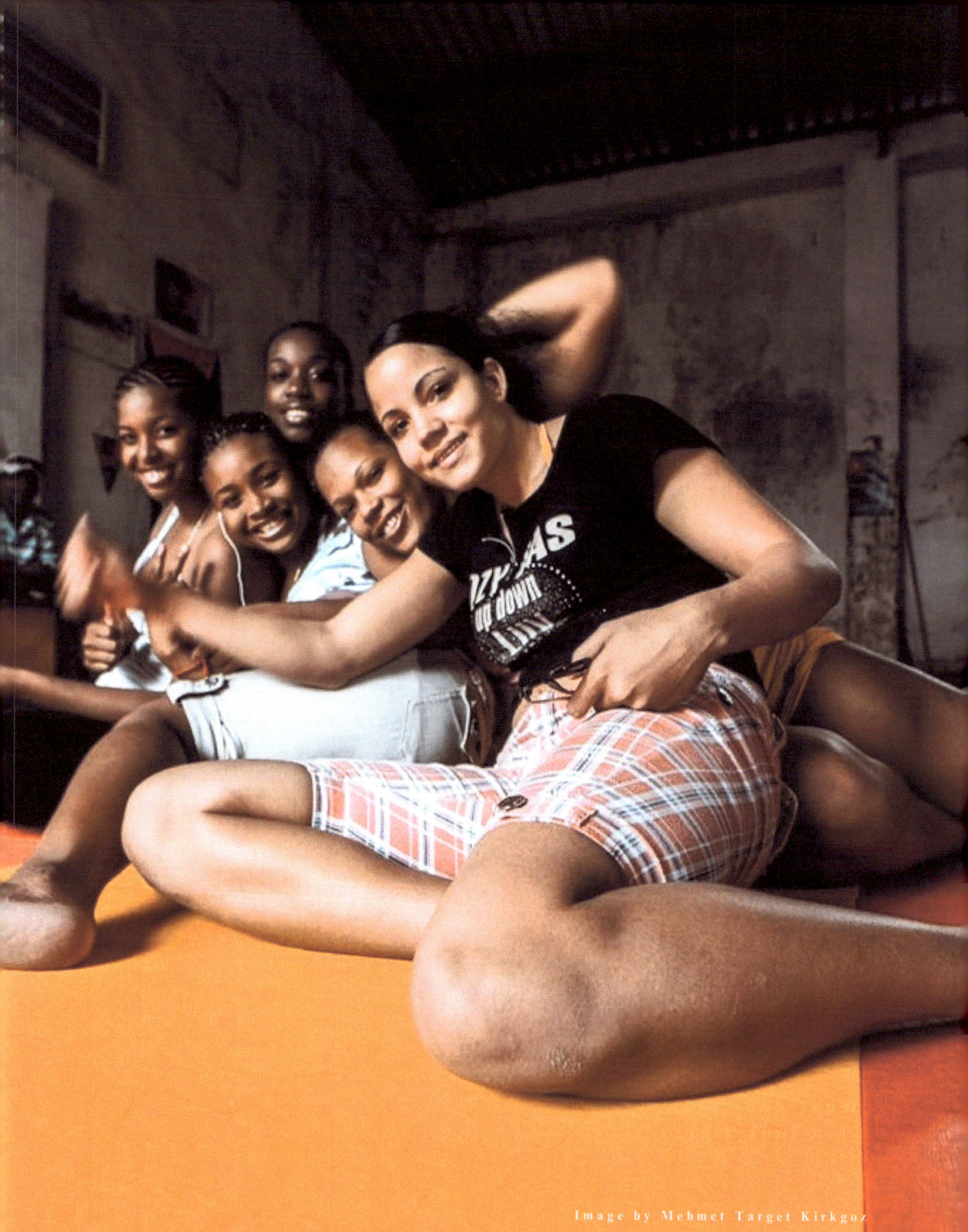

Image by Mehmet Target Kirkgoz

Joining a martial arts class or team has countless benefits:

·Accountability:
Your training partners keep you showing up on days you'd rather stay home.

·Encouragement:
They recognise your progress, even when you overlook it.

·Shared growth:
As they improve, you improve—it's a cycle that pushes everyone forward.

What's even better? The connections formed often go beyond the dojo. It's that group chat full of memes and motivation, or teammates who show up to your belt test to cheer you on.

HERE'S A QUICK TIP: PARTICIPATE IN EVENTS YOUR GROUP ORGANISES, WHETHER IT'S A SEMINAR, FRIENDLY COMPETITION, OR EVEN A BBQ. THESE GATHERINGS STRENGTHEN BONDS, SO IT'S EASIER TO REACH OUT FOR HELP WHEN YOU NEED IT.

Connecting with others reminds you that martial arts is as much about teamwork as it is about personal discipline. You're not just learning skills; you're joining a family.

Reframe mistakes as opportunities and let the people around you soften the edges of your self-criticism.

With mentorship and camaraderie, you'll not only silence that inner critic—you'll thrive.

Being kinder to myself isn't just a nice idea—it's the backbone of my progress. When I stop hammering myself over every misstep, I actually notice all the little victories that fuel my growth.

Letting go of perfection doesn't mean settling; it means building myself up through encouragement and realistic goals.

Progress doesn't happen in an instant—it's made up of small wins and everyday effort. Growth feels lighter when I'm on my own side.

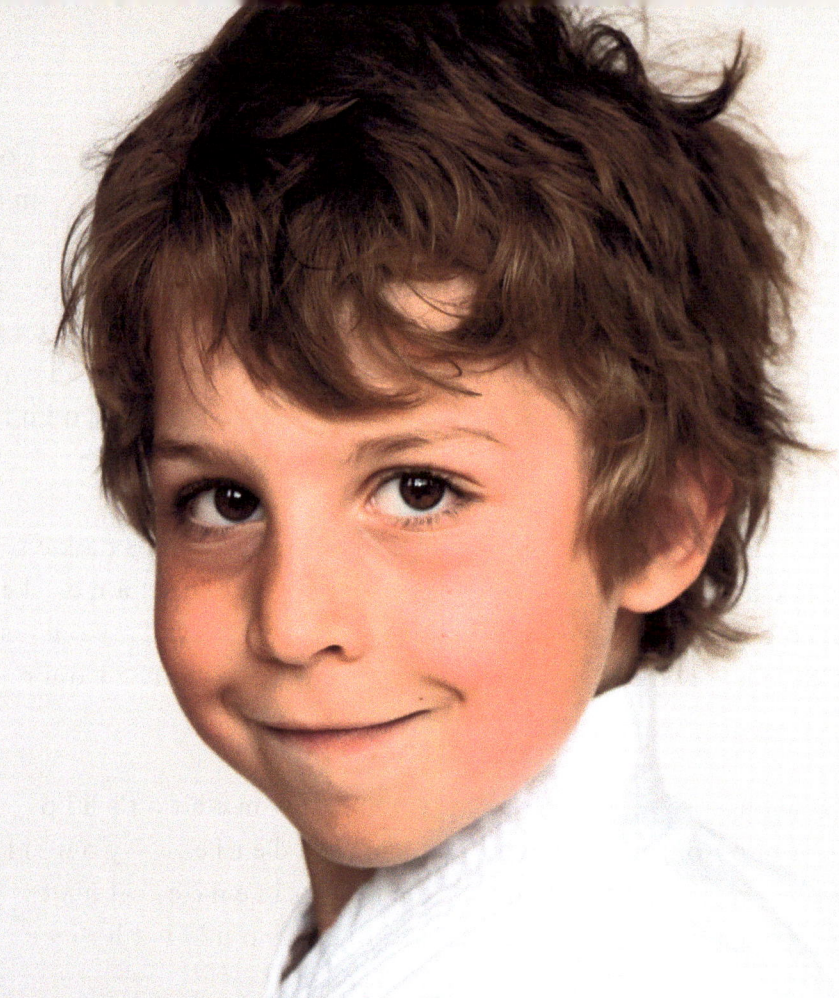

Everybody has a Story to Tell...

AWMA WRITING COMPETITION
Celebrating a Decade of Martial Arts Excellence

Opens February 1st 2025 Closes May 31st 2025

We're excited to announce a special writing competition as part of Albury Wodonga Martial Arts 10th anniversary celebrations!

Whether you're a martial artist or passionate about the martial arts world, this is your opportunity to share your voice while support-ing a worthy cause.

Your Martial Arts Story

Do you have a compelling martial arts tale to tell? Perhaps insights about your training journey? Or thoughtful perspectives on martial arts philosophy? We welcome both fiction and non-fiction entries that celebrate and respect the martial arts tradition.

Your piece could be:

- A creative story featuring martial arts themes
- A personal essay about your training experiences
- An exploration of martial arts philosophy or history
- A reflection on what martial arts means to you

Categories and Prizes

The competition features three age categories with impressive prize pools:

Open (16 and above)
- First Prize: $200 plus 2 year digital subscription to MAMA
- Second Prize: $100 plus 2 year digital subscription
- Third Prize: $50 plus 2 year digital subscription

Maximum word count: 1,000
Entry fee: $10

Youth (10-15 years)

- First Prize: $100 Harvey Norman Gift Voucher plus 2 year digital subscription

- Second Prize: $50 plus 2 year digital subscription

- Third Prize: $25 plus 2 year digital subscription

Maximum word count: 750

Entry fee: $5

Junior (9 years & under)

- First Prize: $100 plus 2 year digital subscription

- Second Prize: $50 plus 2 year digital subscription

- Third Prize: $25 plus 2 year digital subscription

Maximum word count: 750
Entry fee: $5

Special Local Award

For entrants who can attend classes in Wodonga or Beechworth, there's an additional prize of six weeks of free classes with AWMA. Winners can either use this prize themselves or gift it to someone else!

Our Judging Panel

Your work will be evaluated by an expert panel including:

Vanessa McKay, Publications Manager of Martial Arts Magazine Australia

Noah Legel, Renshi 4th Dan, Owner of Illinois Practical Karate

Justin Colbert, Renshi 5th Dan, Owner of Albury Wodonga Martial Arts

Community

This competition isn't just about celebrating martial arts — it's about making a difference. Proceeds will benefit Yes Unlimited, a local organisation with over 40 years of experience supporting young people, those experiencing homelessness, and families escaping domestic violence.

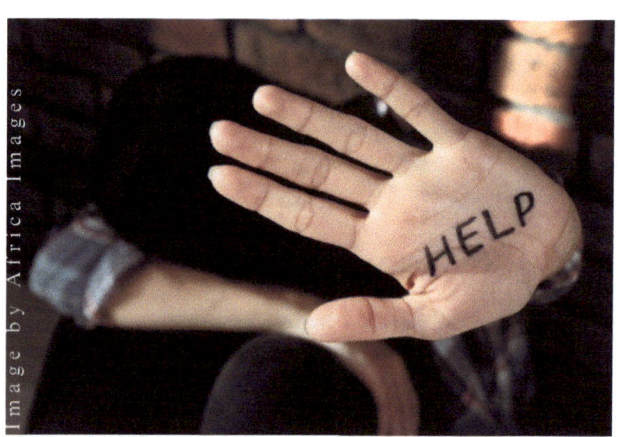
Image by Africa Images

Key Dates

Opens: February 1st, 2025
Closes: May 31st, 2025 12pm (AEST)

Winners announced July 2025 during AWMA's birthday celebrations

Important Guidelines

Entries must be original work (no AI generated content)

Previously unpublished works only

Submit in Microsoft Word format (.doc or .docx)

Double spaced, 11 or 12pt font

Include title and word count at the top

No personal identification details on the submission itself

Entries must be primarily in English

Ready to Enter?

Submit your entry to awmacompetition@gmail.com. Winning entries will be published in Martial Arts Magazine Australia, offering a fantastic opportunity to share your work with the martial arts community.

Don't miss this chance to be part of AWMA's 10th anniversary celebrations while supporting a worthy cause. Grab your keyboard and start writing – we can't wait to read your martial arts story!

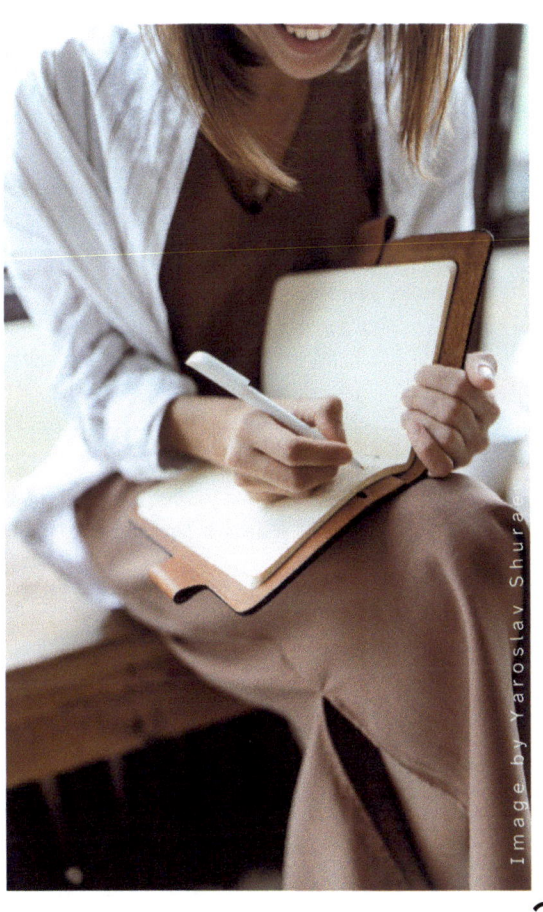

Image by Yaroslav Shuraev

ENTRY FORM
ENTRIES CLOSE 31st of May, 2025

(Print, sign and email to awmacompetition@gmail.com)

NAME	
TITLE OF ENTRY	
ADDRESS	
EMAIL	
PHONE NUMBER	
Optional: DOJO AND RANK/BELT	
CATEGORY: Tick appropriate	☐ OPEN – 16 YEARS AND OLDER ☐ 10 TO 15 YEARS OLD ☐ 9 YEARS OLD AND UNDER ☐ LOCAL (you, or someone you elect, are able to attend classes with AWMA in either Wodonga or Beechworth)
DECLARATION	I have read the terms and conditions and declare that my submission is my original work. _____ Date:___/___/___

Submit to: awmacompetition@gmail.com
Payment details: Jason Colbert BSB 083543 Bank Ac 701102771
  Include the first four letters of your surname + four letters of your story's title
  (For example, your surname is Smith and your story is called "Legend of my Dojo" = SMITLEGE)

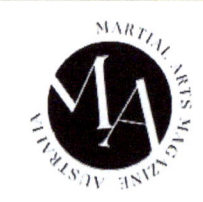
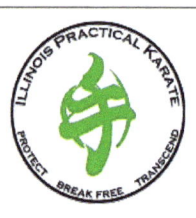

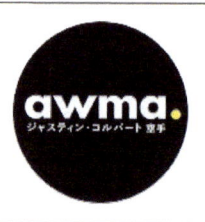

AIKIDO LOVE

BY ATTILA HALASZ

The truth is...
I have visited a few aikido dojos recently and mostly what I saw was...well, "old people" training.

Perhaps the 20-year-olds of today don't have 30 years to master a martial art, like aikido.

But it wasn't always like this. Aikido was popular in the 1990s driven by movies like "Above the Law" and "Hard to Kill" and numerous public demonstrations by various organisations.

Young people flocked to the dojos, and I joined too.

Maybe the pleated hakamas, maybe the art's gentle nature...there were plenty of young ladies drawn to the classes too.

I know a few who met their future partners in the dojo.

This is how I met Mackenzie when I was in my 20s.

I had been doing aikido for a few years when she turned up one day like a beam of sunshine.

Interestingly, we almost instantly noticed each other on the mat.

The white training uniform may not be an attractive piece of clothing, but seeing her in it for the first time, I still thought she is so beautiful!

Pretty and bright, full of laughter and being an artist. When we met, I knew nothing of responsible, healthy eating, but she did.

She introduced me to new ideas, and I did the same for her about things I enjoyed in life. She inspired me and I inspired her and at the next Sydney beach event, we arrived as a couple.

Her best friend was Amelia, who also trained at the dojo. She by chance met a young black belt there named Paul.

Mackenzie and I took it slowly, but Amelia and Paul got married surprisingly soon. Mackenzie made the flower arrangements for the wedding, and I helped deliver them.

I loved that wedding, held in a Spanish-looking building in Sydney that is still there today. I pass the Residencia about twice a year when I'm heading north towards the Central Coast.

"You should be able to read your attacker's energy, their ki that shows their intention. You can then bring their energy into your world and transform that into a peaceful outcome." Said master Ken during one class.

I particularly liked that he was teaching life philosophy and technical stuff.

I understood recognising the opponent's intention is more important than the response itself.

Sure, as Paul and I were both promising black belts at Shin Sen Dojo, we should be able to manifest and implement this according to circumstance.

Except to recognise that Paul's marriage to Amelia was over in a flash. It took eight months to fall apart.

By then Mackenzie and I lived happily together.

Suddenly I noticed Amelia was coming over, more and more. Mostly talking quietly with Mackenzie on the couch. Sometimes she looked distraught.

They would not include me, but I found out from Mackenzie that she wanted out. She thought with marriage, "everything gets better" but them living together showed the opposite.

I was a fool.
When I thought this had nothing to do with me.

One night, she came over with Paul. They announced they were filing for divorce.

Amelia then excitedly told us she was heading to Byron Bay for a fresh start and to join the art and culture community.

...and this will be with her best friend Mackenzie!

Gobsmacked, I sat, but I was told that I could also go along with them if I wanted to!

What? How is this happening?

Until then I was saving up, so I could travel to Paris...together with my girlfriend!

Not to mention there was no way I could leave my established life in Sydney so suddenly.

Only a few weeks later the two women got into a Holden and drove north. My relationship was over.

Even worse, now that Paul had nowhere to live...he moved in with me.

Two sad, idiot black belts who couldn't recognise timely warnings from life and the astonishing change towards uncomfortable energies.

We couldn't see the storm coming. Life demoted us to white belts.

Things felt gloomy.

Heartbreaking, to say the least. Unbelievable by then, but I was going to pop the question in Paris. Even bought a ring in Double Bay.

Paul often rang Amelia about divorce proceedings. One night we were having the usual brown rice dinner.

"I heard Mackenzie has a new guy now...some surfer," Paul told me.

The knife and fork trembled in my hands. Secretly, I hoped she'd come back to me. Against my sanity, I rang her.

"Oh...no, we're just friends...nothing serious," she assured me.

Mackenzie was happy and casual as she spoke.

I hung up the phone and went out to the balcony and sighed.

Paul was there smoking with a beer in hand.

"My heart is broken…she probably slept with the guy. You don't care what Amelia is doing?" I asked. He shrugged his shoulders.

"I'm divorcing," he said.

The proper dagger of words, stabbing right through my heart, came three days later.

The phone rang. Amelia was calling, looking for Paul.

"What is he like…that surfer?" I made the mistake of asking her.

"Josh? He is very cool, he is like an older guy, I think late thirties. He makes McKenzie really happy. He moved in with us a week ago. They are at it all the time, like I have to walk the dog three times a day!" She said.

I never really liked her, but after this, that feeling was definitely cemented!

"Amelia has done you a favour…now you can really move on," Paul said to me with a wry smile. I had to realise that the Mackenzie ship had sailed.

I first thought of a pointless 'revenge' relationship but reading Macrobiotic teacher, George Ohsawa's book had changed my mind. The solution didn't lie there.

I started training even harder instead. Formed a small and dedicated Budo aikido group to complement regular dojo training in a nearby park.

Paul, trained less and less and became more and more withdrawn. To my surprise, many dojo misfits joined me in the park for training.

Rolling, throwing, falling on the grass, with or without weapons and meanwhile keeping our defence effective.

A couple of weeks later, a new student approached me after class.

"I heard about you guys. Can I join you in the park?" She enquired.

Her name was Stella. She had a Mediterranean look with rich black hair. Smaller build, slender and really athletic.

"Are you sure you want to come? Out there the training is intense and hard," I said.

"That's why I'm interested," she smiled.

She joined us the next day.

Locks, pins, hip throws, high falls, she went through it all like a leopard with ferocious spirit. She earned her place and our respect. This tiny but enthusiastic outdoor group really made a difference to our aikido training.

I kept inviting Paul, but he declined and worked from home a lot instead.

After a sweaty and powerful training in the park, Stella turned to me:

"I'll have to head into the city for a job interview this evening at a restaurant. Since you live close by, can I take a shower and get ready at your place?"

"Sure...happy to help with anything."

We walked home wearing our aikido uniforms.

I introduced Stella quickly to Paul, and she went to shower, change clothes and get interview ready.

When she reappeared, she was quite a sight!

Polished black ankle boots with shiny stockings, she wore a high fashion beige miniskirt and an elegantly crisp, skinny fit white top.

Autumn lipstick and frizzled hair completed this stunning picture.

"I'm so nervous about this job. I really need it. Can I have a cigarette?" She asked Paul.

A minute later, they both sat on the balcony, smoking and talking.

(Most people at aikido didn't smoke, but those two did!)

Paul, the self-imposed recluse, suddenly became an outgoing and fun conversationalist.

Half an hour later, Stella rushed off to the interview.

I agreed to put her aikido uniform in the wash and bring it to the next dojo class for her.

Later, as I was cooking dinner in the kitchen, Paul came by leaning against the door frame.

"So...when is the next outdoor training?" he asked.

While cooking the brown rice, I smiled.

Paul came to the classes and Stella became a frequent visitor at our place. Her positive presence transformed Paul.

When Stella arrived, Paul acted and looked like... he was waiting for her all his life!

Notably, she was her own proud woman, and her incredibly inspiring spirit captivated Paul.

Paul became this new person I had never seen before.

She too had the biggest smile every time she saw Paul arriving at class. Everything felt natural and fitting for them from the moment they touched.

I am still proud that I had something to do with them meeting each other. For those two, everything was well in the aikido universe.

Real love cannot be stopped.

It was almost two years later in 1996 when Paul rang me.

"I'm getting married," he said with his voice beaming.

"Am I going to be the best man?" I asked.

"Yes!" he said.

An amazing wedding followed in the Blue Mountains. Only this time, it felt to be the right one.

Many guests from the aikido dojo attended.

Today Stella and Paul live happily married in Canberra. They have two beautiful, now grown-up children.

They don't do aikido anymore...probably because they don't need to.

Those training in aikido probably already know, this great martial art helps you outside the tatami more. It can actually guide you through life.

I know, you wonder. But what of me? Did I miss out on my aikido love?

Twenty-nine years since we've met I can report that I too found the love of my life, in circumstances that you wouldn't believe. But that's another story to tell.

by Attila Halasz
Instagram: aikido.guardian

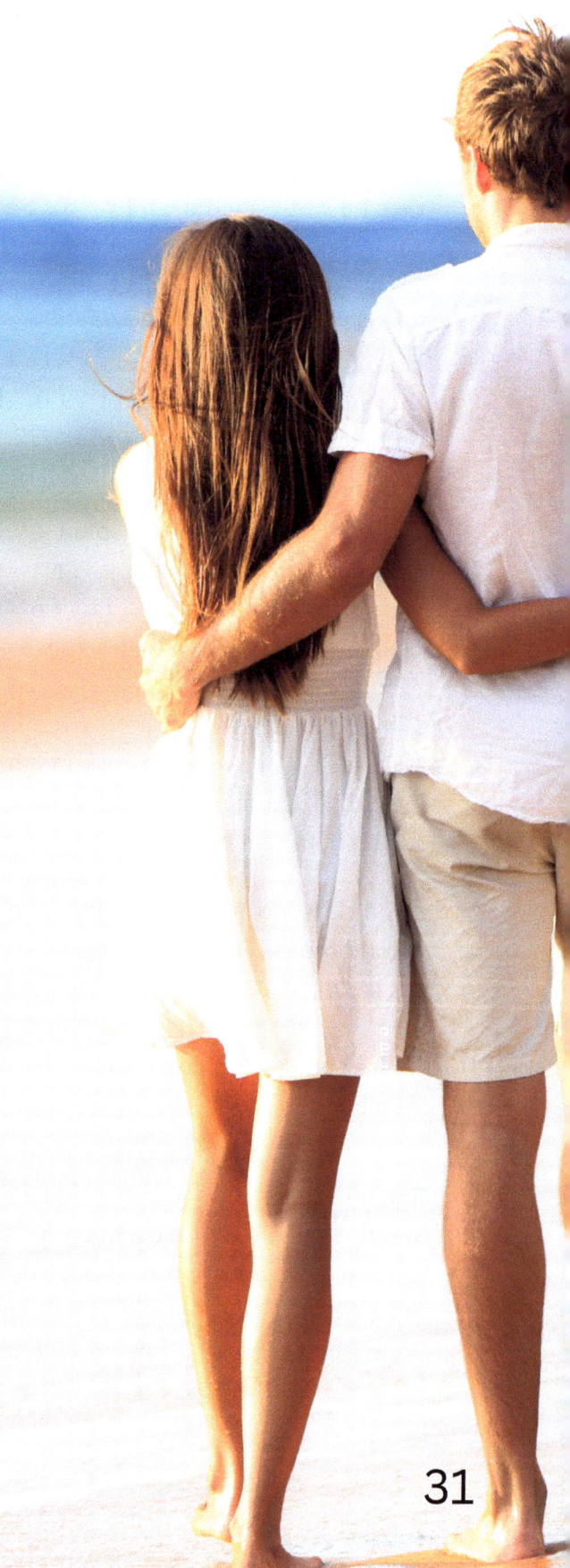

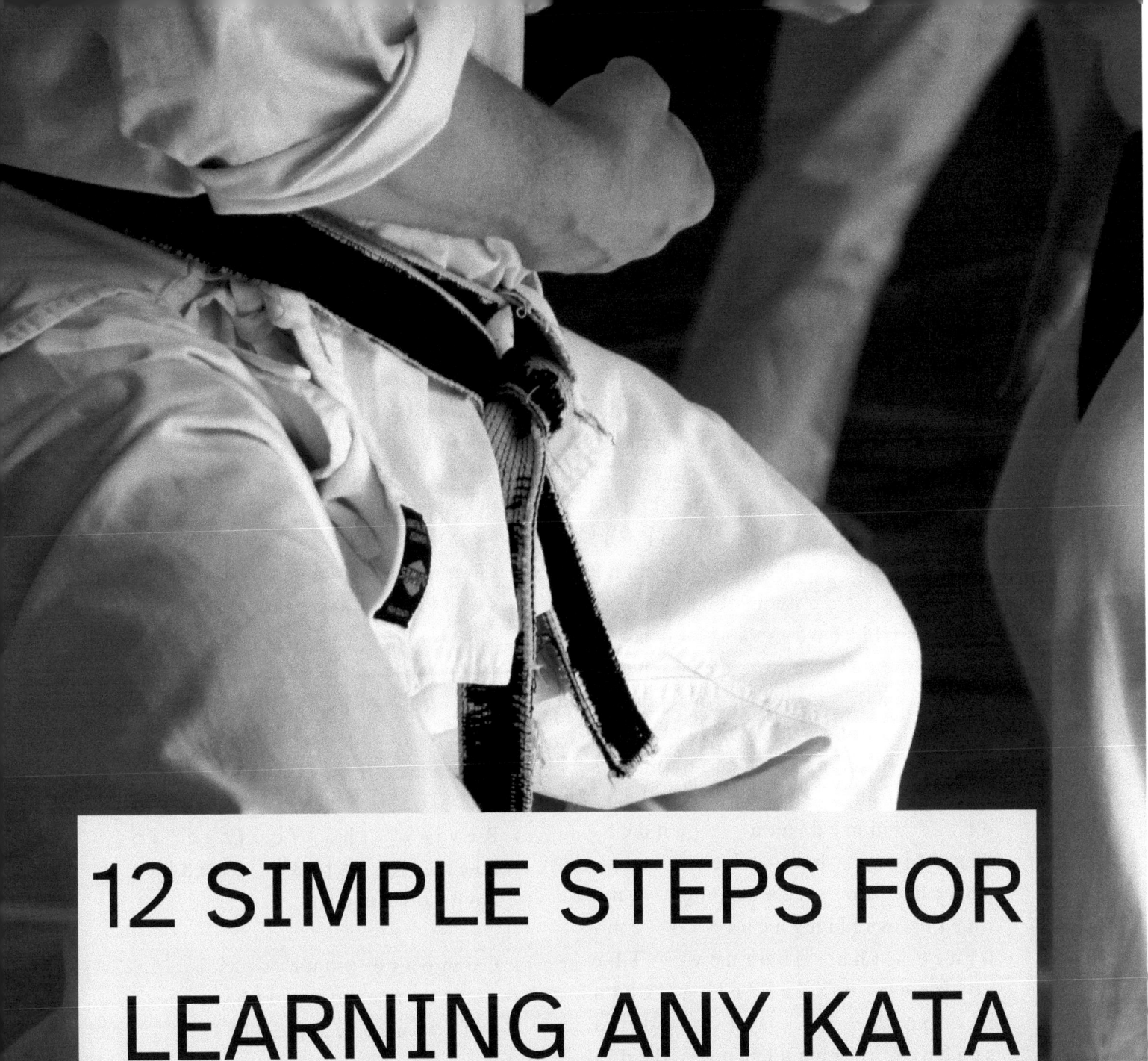

12 SIMPLE STEPS FOR LEARNING ANY KATA

By Don McKay

Standing in the dojo, facing a new kata for the first time, it's natural to feel a mix of excitement and apprehension. Many practitioners find themselves worried about making mistakes, feeling self-conscious about their coordination, or concerned they won't grasp the sequence quickly enough. These feelings are a completely normal part of the learning process - even the most accomplished martial artists were once beginners who had to learn their first kata. What sets successful practitioners apart isn't natural talent or immediate understanding, but their approach to learning and their willingness to embrace the journey. The journey of learning kata is both an art and a science, requiring dedication, patience, and systematic practice.

Lets summarise twelve proven methods for learning kata, each offering a different pathway to understanding kata. These techniques can be combined and adapted to suit your individual learning style.

Step-by-Step Breakdown
- Start by learning the basic sequence without power or speed
- Break the kata into smaller sections or combinations
- Practice each section until you can perform it smoothly before moving to the next
- Gradually connect the sections together

Video Recording
- Record yourself performing the kata
- Review the footage to identify areas needing improvement
- Compare your performance with reference examples

Follow Along Learning
- Train with someone who performs the movements while you follow
- Use video resources as supplementary aids at home

- Focus on getting the general pattern first before refining details

Mirror Training
- Practice in front of a mirror to check your form
- Pay attention to stance details, hand positions, and overall alignment
- Use the mirror to spot and correct common mistakes

Line by Line Method
- Learn the kata by directional changes or "lines" of movement
- Master each directional sequence before moving to the next
- Focus on proper turning and transitional movements

Application Based Learning (Bunkai)
- Learn the practical applications of each movement as you learn them
- Understanding the purpose helps you to memorise the sequence
- Practice with a partner to better grasp the techniques

Visualisation Techniques
- Mentally rehearse the kata
- Create memory aids like counting patterns or movement sequences
- Visualise opponents' positions and attacks

Pattern Walking
- Practice the footwork pattern, no techniques
- Focus on doing proper stances and transitions
- Add upper body movements when you have memorised the kata

Slow Motion Practice
- Perform the entire kata in slow motion
- Focus on perfect form and breathing

- Gradually increase speed as proficiency improves

Teaching Others

- Explaining the kata to others helps reinforce your understanding

- Break down complex movements for others

- Answer questions about details you might have overlooked

Kata Journalling

- Maintain a timeline of your kata progression by documenting each training session with specific details about what you practiced, challenges encountered, and breakthroughs you experienced.

- Create detailed breakdowns of each kata section. Write notes on stance details, hand positions, weight and breathing patterns.

- Use your journal to track feedback and corrections from your instructors.

Kata Mapping

- This spatial tool helps students to understand the overall flow and rhythm of the kata.

- Gain deeper insights into the internal mechanics and energy flow of the kata.

- Map out an attackers angles, and defensive responses to transform abstract movements into meaningful applications.

Learning a new kata is a journey that becomes more rewarding as you develop your own unique approach to mastering these traditional forms. The twelve methods outlined above aren't meant to be used in isolation - rather, they form a toolkit from which you can select and combine techniques that resonate with your learning style. Some days you might focus on slow-motion practice and visualization, while others might call for pattern walking and mirror training.

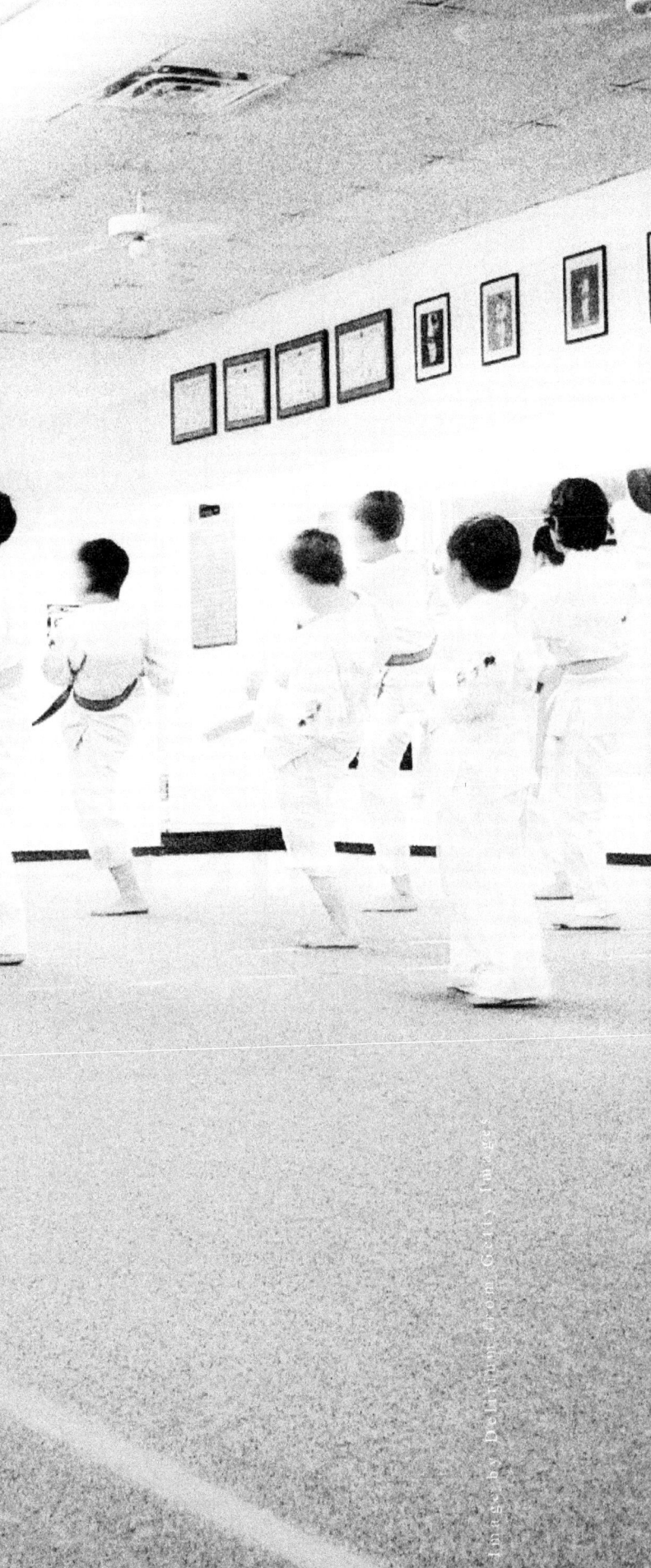

Remember that every martial artist's journey is different. What works best for one practitioner might not be the optimal approach for another. The key is to remain patient with yourself and maintain consistency in your practice. Start with methods that feel most natural to you, then gradually incorporate others as your confidence grows. Through regular practice and the systematic application of these learning techniques, you'll find that even the most complex kata become accessible and meaningful.

Most importantly, don't be afraid to make mistakes along the way - they're an essential part of the learning process. Each training session, whether it feels successful or challenging, contributes to your growth as a martial artist. Trust in the process, stay dedicated to your practice, and remember that every master once stood where you stand now, learning their first kata one step at a time.

Don McKay
KarateforLife.net

BEAT THE HEAT THIS SUMMER

Image from ImageStock by Getty

The Australian summer presents unique challenges for martial artists, with temperatures regularly soaring above 35°C in many regions. This guide explores how to maintain effective training while staying safe during the scorching summer months.

The Australian Climate

The Australian summer, typically running from December to February, brings intense heat, high humidity in coastal regions, and prolonged periods of extreme temperatures. Unlike more temperate climates, our summers can see consecutive days above 40°C, making traditional martial arts training methods potentially dangerous without proper modification.

Hydration

Proper hydration is crucial when training in Australian conditions. The body loses fluids rapidly through sweating, particularly when training in a gi.

Before Training:
- Drink 600ml of water in the two hours before training.
- Include electrolyte drinks if training will exceed 45 minutes.
- Avoid caffeine and alcohol in the hours leading up to training.
- Monitor urine colour - pale yellow indicates good hydration.

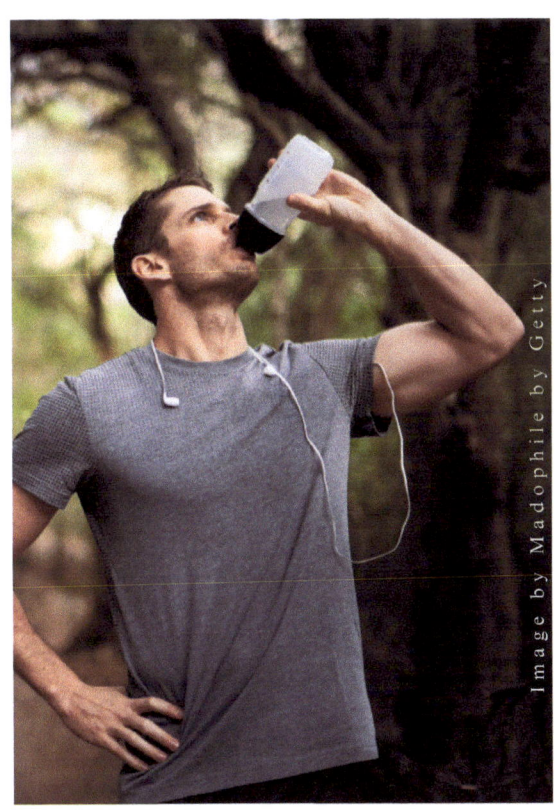

During Training:
- Keep water bottle within easy reach.
- Take small sips every 10 15 minutes.
- Aim for 200 - 250ml every 15 minutes.

- Consider sports drinks for sessions longer than an hour.
- Don't wait until you're thirsty. That's already too late.

After Training:

- ·Weigh yourself before and after training to gauge fluid loss.
- ·Drink 1.5 times the amount of fluid lost through sweat.
- ·Include electrolyte rich foods in post training meals.
- ·Continue hydrating for several hours after training.

Examples of Electrolyte Rich Foods

- **Sodium-rich foods:** table and sea salt, pickled vegetables, seaweed, miso soup, cottage cheese, wholemeal bread, tinned soup, salted nuts.
- **Potassium-rich foods:** bananas, sweet potatoes, white potatoes skin on, spinach, yoghurt, avocados, coconut water, rock melon, dried apricots.
- **Magnesium-rich foods:** dark leafy greens, pumpkin seeds, almonds, black beans, tofu, dark chocolate, brown rice, quinoa, chia seeds.
- **Calcium-rich foods:** dairy products, sardines with bones, fortified plant milks, bok choy, kale, broccoli, figs, tahini.
- **Chloride-rich foods:** celery, tomatoes, lettuce, olives, seaweed.

Easy Pre/Post Training Snack Ideas:

- Banana with a handful of salted nuts.
- Yoghurt with fruit and seeds.
- Smoothie made with coconut water and spinach.
- Apple slices with nut butter.
- Rice crackers with avocado.
- Trail mix with dried fruit and nuts.
- Homemade sports drink (coconut water, pinch of salt, lemon juice).

Remember that timing of these foods is important - eat easily digestible options before training and save heavier foods for post-training recovery.

Heat Related Illness

The Australian summer demands vigilance in monitoring yourself and your training partners for signs of heat related illness. Here are the key symptoms to watch for:

Heat Exhaustion:
- Heavy sweating
- Cool, clammy skin
- Weakness or fatigue
- Dizziness or headache
- Nausea
- Rapid, shallow breathing
- Muscle cramps

Heat Stroke (Medical Emergency):
- Cessation of sweating
- Hot, dry skin
- Confusion/disorientation
- Severe headache
- Temperature above 40°C
- Rapid, strong pulse
- Loss of consciousness

Action for Heat Related Illness

1. Stop all physical activity
2. Move to a cool, space
3. Remove excess clothing,
4. Apply cool, wet towels to neck, armpits, and groin
5. Sip water slowly don't gulp
6. If symptoms of heat stroke appear, call 000 immediately
7. Use ice packs if available
8. Fan the person
9. Monitor vital signs until help arrives

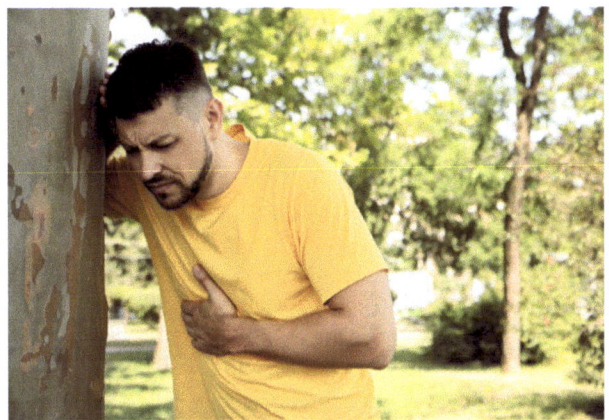

Training Modifications
Adapting your training approach becomes essential during the summer months:

Timing and Location:
- Schedule training for early morning or evening.
- Utilise indoor, air-conditioned dojos where possible.

- If training outdoors, seek shaded areas.
- Consider moving certain training elements to swimming pools.

Gi and Equipment:
- Invest in lightweight, breathable gi material.
- Keep a spare gi for changing if necessary.
- Consider training in rash guards for certain sessions.
- Use sweat bands to prevent sweat affecting vision.
- Keep equipment clean and dry to prevent bacterial growth.

Training Structure:
- Extend warm up periods to accommodate the heat.
- Include more frequent water breaks.
- Reduce high intensity intervals.
- Focus on technique rather than power.
- Modify kata practice to manage exertion levels.
- Incorporate more paired technical work.
- Reduce sparring duration and intensity.

Using the Heat

While the summer heat presents challenges, it also offers opportunities for specific training benefits:

Flexibility Enhancement:
- Warmer muscles allow for greater stretching potential.
- Use the natural heat to improve high kicks.
- Focus on mobility work during peak heat.
- Incorporate dynamic stretching sequences.

Technical Refinement:
- Slower, more deliberate movement practice.
- Focus on stance work and transitions.
- Perfect basic techniques without power.
- Work on breathing co-ordination.
- Develop efficient movement patterns.

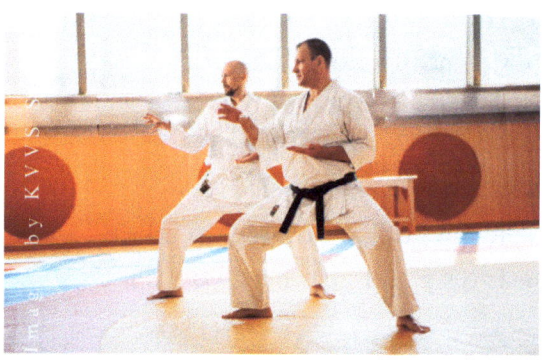

Mental Training:
- Use heat as a tool for developing mental toughness.
- Practice meditation and breathing exercises.
- Work on visualisation techniques.
- Develop heat tolerance gradually.

Nutrition

Proper nutrition becomes even more critical during summer training.

Before Training:
- Light, easily digestible meals 2 - 3 hours before.
- Fresh fruits for natural hydration.
- Complex carbohydrates for sustained energy.
- Avoid heavy proteins immediately before training.

During Training:
- Small amounts of fruit if needed.
- Sports gels for longer sessions.
- Electrolyte replacement drinks.

After Training:
- Potassium rich foods (bananas, sweet potatoes)
- Lean proteins for muscle recovery.
- Magnesium rich foods to prevent cramping.
- Replace salt with food or sports drinks.

Recovery Strategies
- Enhanced recovery protocols help maintain training consistency through summer:

Cooling Methods
- Cool showers or ice baths.
- Cold towels on neck and head.
- Use of cooling fans.
- Gentle walking to gradually lower body temperature.

Rest and Recovery:
- Increased sleep during hot periods.
- Active recovery sessions in air-conditioned spaces.
- Pool recovery sessions.
- Gentle stretching in cool environments.

Environmental Concerns

Managing your training environment becomes crucial:

Indoor Training:
- Ensure proper ventilation.
- Use fans strategically.
- Monitor humidity levels
- Keep training areas clean and dry.
- Have backup cooling options available.

Outdoor Training:
- Check weather forecasts and UV indexes.
- Plan around extreme heat days.
- ·Have shade options available.
- Consider training on grass rather than concrete.
- Keep first aid supplies readily accessible.

Special Considerations for Children and Seniors

Extra care must be taken with vulnerable groups:

Children:
- More frequent water breaks.
- Shorter training segments.
- Closer monitoring for heat stress.
- Modified uniform requirements.
- Enhanced supervision during summer months.

Seniors:
- Adjusted training intensities.
- More gradual warmups.
- Regular temperature hecks.
- Modified training times
- Enhanced hydration protocols.

Emergency Readiness

Emergency protocols are essential:

- First aid kit specifically for heat related issues: digital thermometer to monitor body temperature
- Multiple instant cold packs (chemical activation type), reusable ice packs (keep frozen in nearby freezer)
- Several clean spray bottles for misting water, electrolyte replacement powder/tablets, oral rehydration solutions (like Hydralyte)
- Clean towels of varying sizes, Emergency thermal blankets (can be used to reflect heat)

- Cooling neck wraps or bandanas.
- Sponges for cooling.
- Emergency contact numbers are visible.
- Cooling equipment is readily available.
- Trained first aid responders present.

Know your limits

Understand and assess your personal heat tolerance:

Monitor Your Signals:
- Track how you feel during training at different temperatures.
- Note when you start feeling uncomfortable or fatigued.
- Record your heart rate response to exertion in heat.
- Document any symptoms like dizziness, nausea, or headaches.
- Pay attention to how quickly you recover after heat exposure.

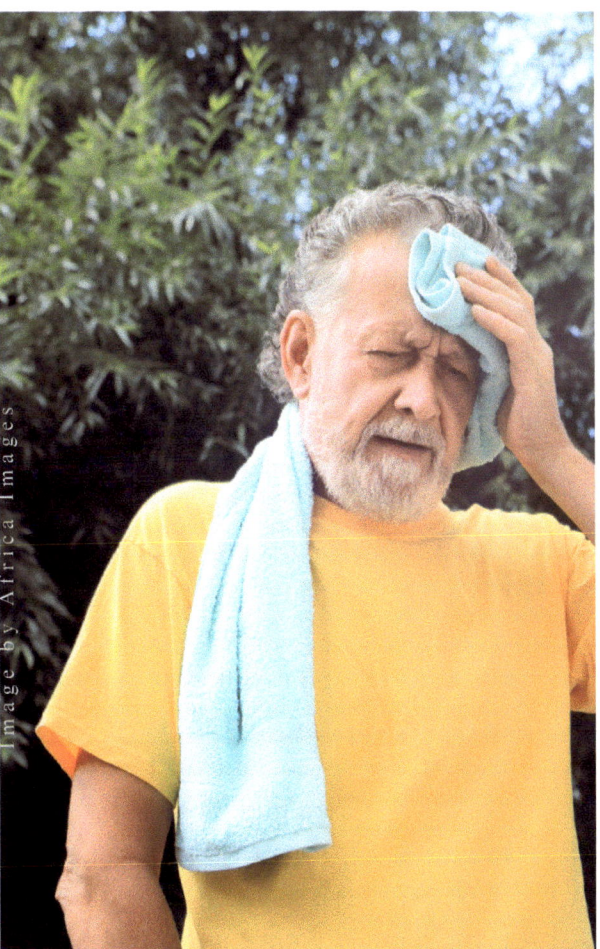

- Monitor your vital signs and comfort level.
- Gradually increase duration and intensity.
- Keep a log of temperature, humidity, and your response.
- Note your performance decline thresholds.

Gradual Testing Method:
- Start with short sessions (15-20 mins) in warm conditions.

Factors That Affect Heat Tolerance:
- ·Fitness level
- ·Age
- ·Body composition

44

- Medical conditions.
- Medications.
- Hydration status.
- Recent illness/fatigue.
- Acclimatisation level.

Warning Signs You've Reached Your Limit:

- Difficulty maintaining normal training pace.
- Excessive sweating or sudden stop in sweating.
- Mental confusion or difficulty concentrating.
- Muscle cramping.
- Rapid heartbeat that doesn't settle with rest.
- Feeling unusually tired or weak.
- Headache or dizziness
- Nausea.

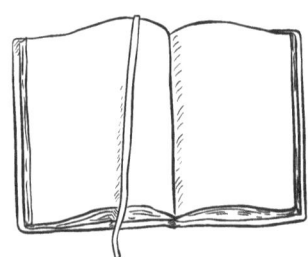

Practical Assessment:

1. Use a diary to record:
- Temperature and humidity.
- Duration of activity
- Intensity level.
- How you felt during and after.
- Recovery time needed.
- Symptoms experienced.

2. Personal heat scale:
- Green zone: Comfortable, can train normally.
- Yellow zone: Need modifications but can continue.
- Red zone: Must stop or significantly modify activity.

Professional Input:

- Consider consulting a sports physician.
- Get a fitness assessment that includes heat stress testing.
- Work with experienced instructors who can monitor your response.
- Consider having basic health metrics checked regularly.

Heat tolerance can change over time and with different circumstances, so it's important to regularly reassess and adjust accordingly.

- Carry your emergency contact information.
- Keep personal medical information available.
- Understand when to stop training.
- Know local emergency services locations.

> **Pure Water is the world's first and foremost medicine.**
>
> SLOVAKIAN PROVERB

By following these guidelines, you can maintain effective training throughout the summer months while ensuring safety and continued progress in your martial arts journey. Remember that adapting to conditions shows wisdom rather than weakness, and maintaining consistent, safe training through summer will lead to better long-term development in your martial arts practice.

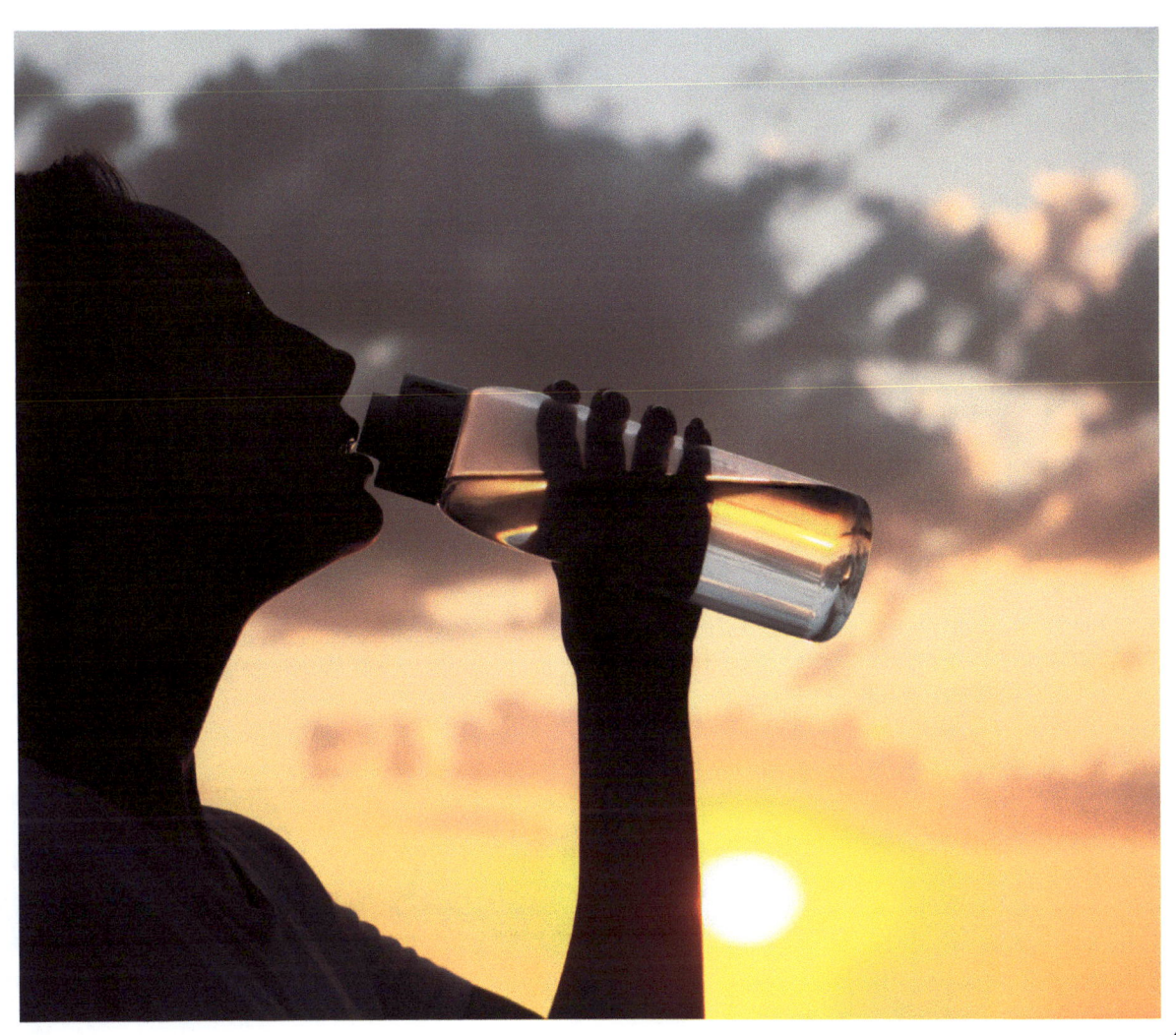

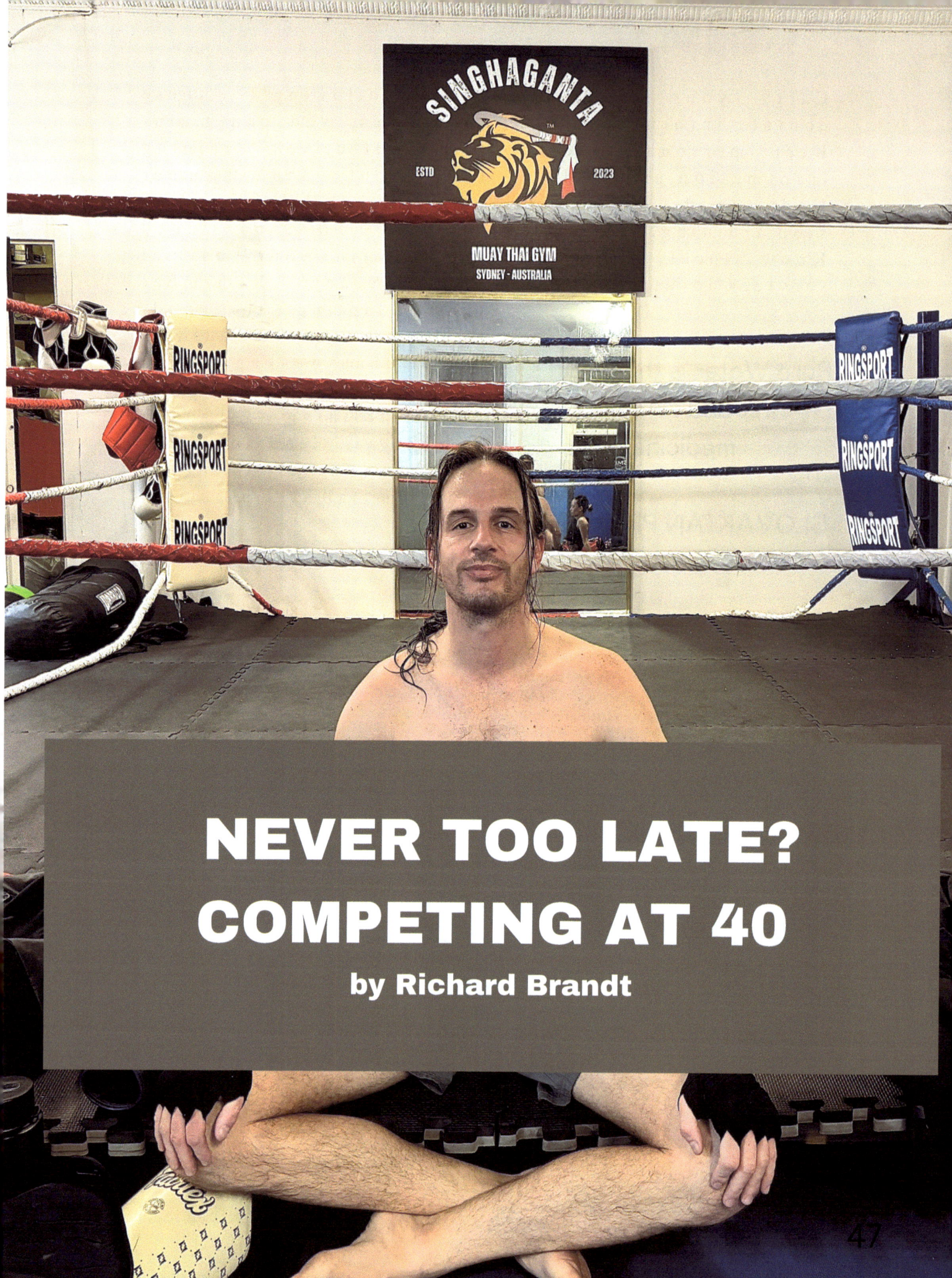

"If you can walk, you can train." Words from legendary trainer Thohsaphol Master Toddy Sitiwatjana in a social media post promoting his Muay Thai camp in Bangkok.

Master Toddy's attitude echoes the adage "age is just a number." He says, "you are never too old" (to start) and guarantees he can find a competition to enrol you in with "whatever you need" regarding protective gear or a suitable opponent. All this had my attention. Partly because Master Toddy's camp has been in my periphery for some time as something I might like to do in the future (my algorithm knows me well). But mostly because I was seeing this post not long after completing my four-hour-per-day training camp on Koh Samui to mark 40 of my own years on Earth.

The idea that competitive sport is a young person's pursuit endures.

Yet in recent years, athletes from various disciplines have succeeded at an elite level well beyond what is traditionally considered prime athletic age. Serena Williams retired from professional tennis at 40. Lewis Hamilton turns 40 in January and is still driving in Formula 1 with at least two years to go. Kelly Slater won the Pipe Masters six days out from his fiftieth birthday in 2022. Many combat athletes, perhaps currently most notably Alex Pereira, are well into their thirties. I acknowledge that these examples are special cases. But why can't this phenomenon trickle down to the amateur leagues? (And let's not forget, at the more mortal end of the spectrum, about Tom Hardy winning a Brazilian Jiu Jitsu competition under a pseudonym at 45 and has since gone on to further wins.) Yet, when asked, almost all my similarly aged peers say the ship has sailed on competitive fighting, even at a club level. Are they doing themselves a disservice?

The idea that competitive sport is a young person's pursuit endures.

At 34, I was what you might call a late starter in martial arts. I started with Krav Maga with the goal of learning self-defence skills and a commitment to myself to endure a minimum of six months of training. Accidentally, I became an instructor in around 20 months. And never did I think my foray into training Muay Thai on the side would morph into a full-time pursuit, resulting in me signing up to participate in an inter-gym exhibition fight.

Our coaches, possessing experience in this scene, really pushed us. Running before class. Two-hour plus sessions five times per week. Harder than usual sparring and for many more rounds per class. I think several of my teammates who were also taking part for the first time were surprised how hard we were being pushed for a friendly inter-gym meet. This was as close to a fight camp as it could be with the limitation of day job and adequate recovery was an abstract concept in the lead-up to the event. I loved all of it.

In a swing of Murphy's Law, I had been unwell during the final lead-up to the day. I was not fully fit on fight day, something I kept to myself, and I almost pulled out. Thinking the Fear of Missing Out would feel worse than anything that would happen in the ring, I chose to push through (as the Thais say, sûu sûu/สู้ๆ!). I still wasn't sure what to expect in terms of the number and length of rounds or the striking intensity. I didn't even know who my opponent was until I met him in the ring. I suspect many of us, like me, were preoccupied pre-fight assessing the crowd for our most likely match-ups based on size, hoping for a more desk worker type than a builder.

Matches were three rounds of 90 seconds each with a 30-second rest between rounds, meaning we could pump through all 27 bouts in half a day. Fighters wore full protective gear, including headgear and a body vest, which I half expected, but honestly would have preferred to do without.

The juniors went first, with the rest of us competing in a random order. My match was just over halfway down the card. Plenty of time then to support a few people ahead of me, while becoming suitably nervous. At one point, the energy became too much and I had to take recess in the breakout room to warm up early, purely to remove myself from the chaotic energy to settle down. This was a lesson in self-management as much as it was in fighting.

In the end, I had less time to prepare than expected as my bout was brought forward by two matches for an unspecified reason. I had joked with some friends before the event that as long as my opponent's not 25, I'll be fine. Sure enough, stepping into the ring I was met by an athletic looking young bloke of a similar size who turned out to be 25 on the dot (it's okay, just sûu sûu!). A touch of gloves and it was on.

While this was billed as a friendly sparring day of exhibition matches for fun and learning purposes, make no mistake, the intensity was very real. Striking was full power. I hadn't worn headgear in probably more than two years and felt like it amplified the heat several degrees (but, thankfully, it kept my long hair which I'm always battling in training out of my face!). The cheers and shouted advice from the crowd just background noise blended with the looped recording of the Sarama. I am still haunted by one of my coaches telling me to check more at the break between the first and second rounds followed by my other coach telling me to try and land some kicks. This wasn't going to happen. My health let me down. My legs like sandbags, my kicks slow. It's all I could do to absorb kicks on my guard and resort to hands for the most part.

The feedback from my teammates was encouraging. Apparently I outboxed my opponent with hands and left no openings for counter punches (thank you Krav Maga boxing training!). An experienced teammate with around ten amateur fights behind him didn't know I was forty and was blown away, showering praise when I told him. Although in reality, if this wasn't an exhibition, I would have lost on account of kicks. I was also swept twice, but landed one sweep of my own. The negative points I already knew and at least my health was the one underlying reason that would fix itself. Plenty of takeaways to work on. The main thing was, it was done.

So how was it? In a word: hard. I was no stranger to challenges in martial arts. I have been crushed by 115 kilogram guys in Brazilian Jiu Jitsu. In Krav Maga I have sparred with ex-military, black belts and high-ranked instructors from other disciplines. For my brown belt test in Krav Maga I passed a four-hour grading partnered with my former instructor-turned-personal protection professional, who outweighs me by about ten kilograms and is built like a racing colt.

Yet this "fight" was harder than anything I had done previously. I think the lies in that while a martial arts grading isn't easy, the outcome is you either pass or fail. Even under pressure during level tests there is never any real danger of lasting consequences since damage causing injury or knock out is not the goal. By contrast, during a competitive round you are in the firing line the entire time. You need to be alert for the duration of a round. A lapse in concentration or a slow reaction could result in a KO. You are balancing survival against putting in a competitive showing yourself. Even preparing for it was harder than any training I had done previously. My respect for what combat sport athletes do went stratospheric following this experience.

Having done another one since it seems these sparring meetings can be a bit Wild West. The talent pool is limited to a few gyms and while the organisers do their best, suitable match-ups with regard to weight and experience can be a bit loose. It was a minor miracle no one was knocked out as some fights descended into all-out brawling. There was the odd injury and a couple of bleeding noses. In hindsight being halfway down the card this was a good thing, as the intensity of these events tend not to follow any kind of bell curve distribution. Rather, as the heat and testosterone increases throughout the event, so too does the excitement along with the intensity of each match at the expense of what I would call quality technique. Ninety seconds is not a lot of time to get any work done, so guys come out of the gates firing like greyhounds chasing a fake rabbit to make an impression.

Competitive martial arts isn't, or shouldn't, be about being the best, the It is about sport and testing yourself and pushing your body and skills in a fair competition. Let's face it, in sport age is a factor. You will age out of a competitive peak sooner or later. But to put a cap on when you can compete based on an arbitrary number is, in my opinion, the result of a limiting belief in oneself. You might be past mixing with teenagers, but what's wrong with that? Everyone has their reasons for starting martial arts and their own motivations to persevere with training. If the reason is fitness or community, that's fine. But if you are serious about being an effective practitioner and have the opportunity, you owe it to yourself to try competing in some capacity at least once whatever your age. Whether it's a masters division in a local tournament or the Golden Gloves (yes, it's real!), just sign up. As many professional athletes show us, if age is no barrier, what's your excuse?

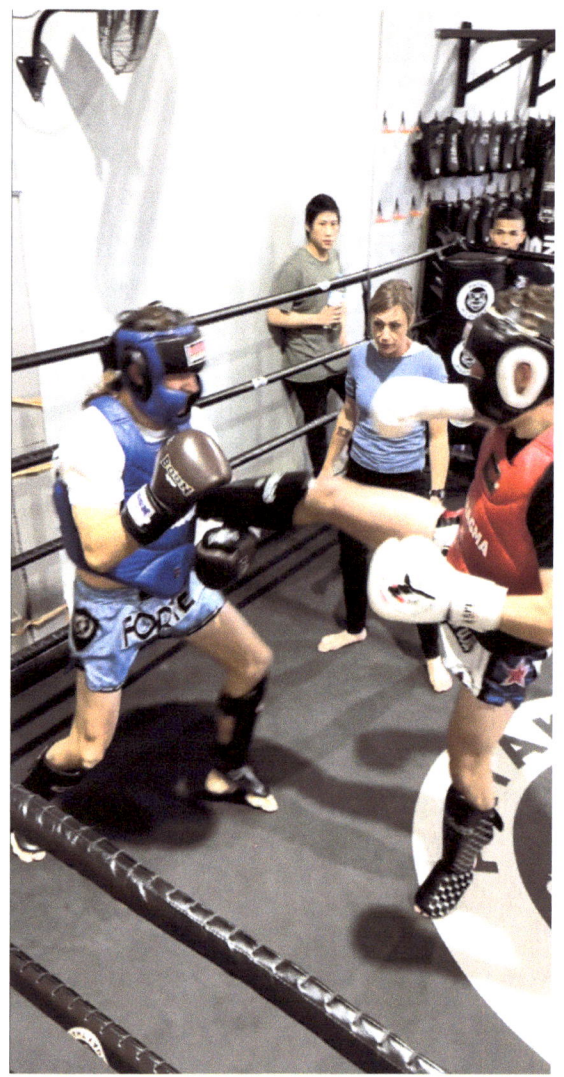

I suppose the next thing for me is to do a fully sanctioned fight complete with judges and a win on the line. I just need to find a suitable promotion.

Maybe I'll give Master Toddy a call.

Richard Brandt is a certified senior Krav Maga instructor and Muay Thai practitioner training out of Singhaganata Muay Thai gym in Sydney. He has trained both disciplines locally, in Israel and all over South-East Asia.

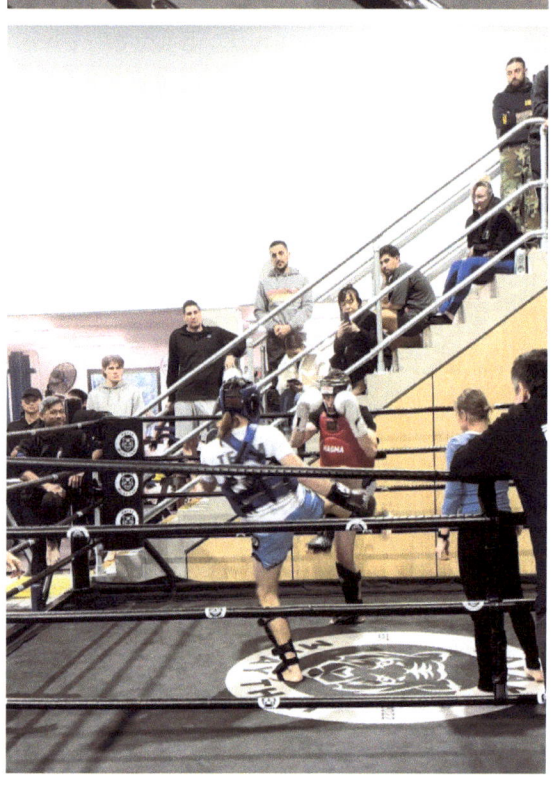

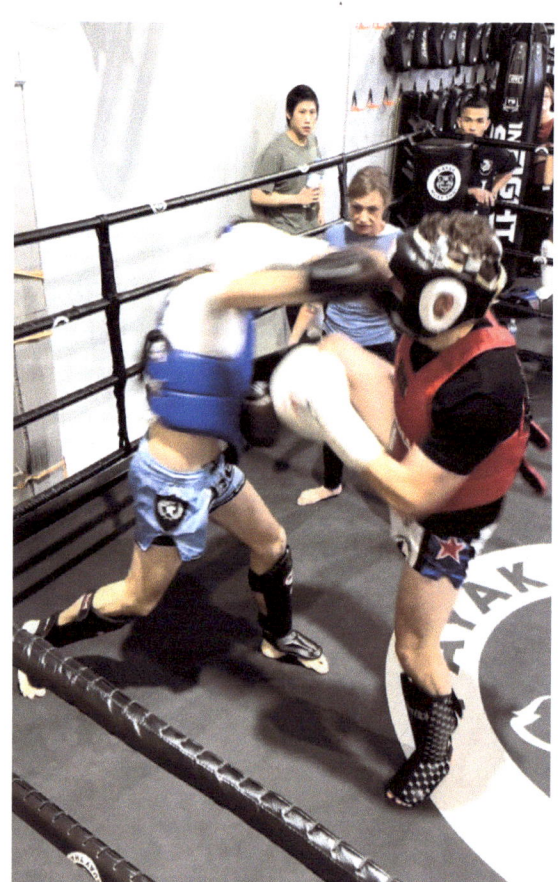

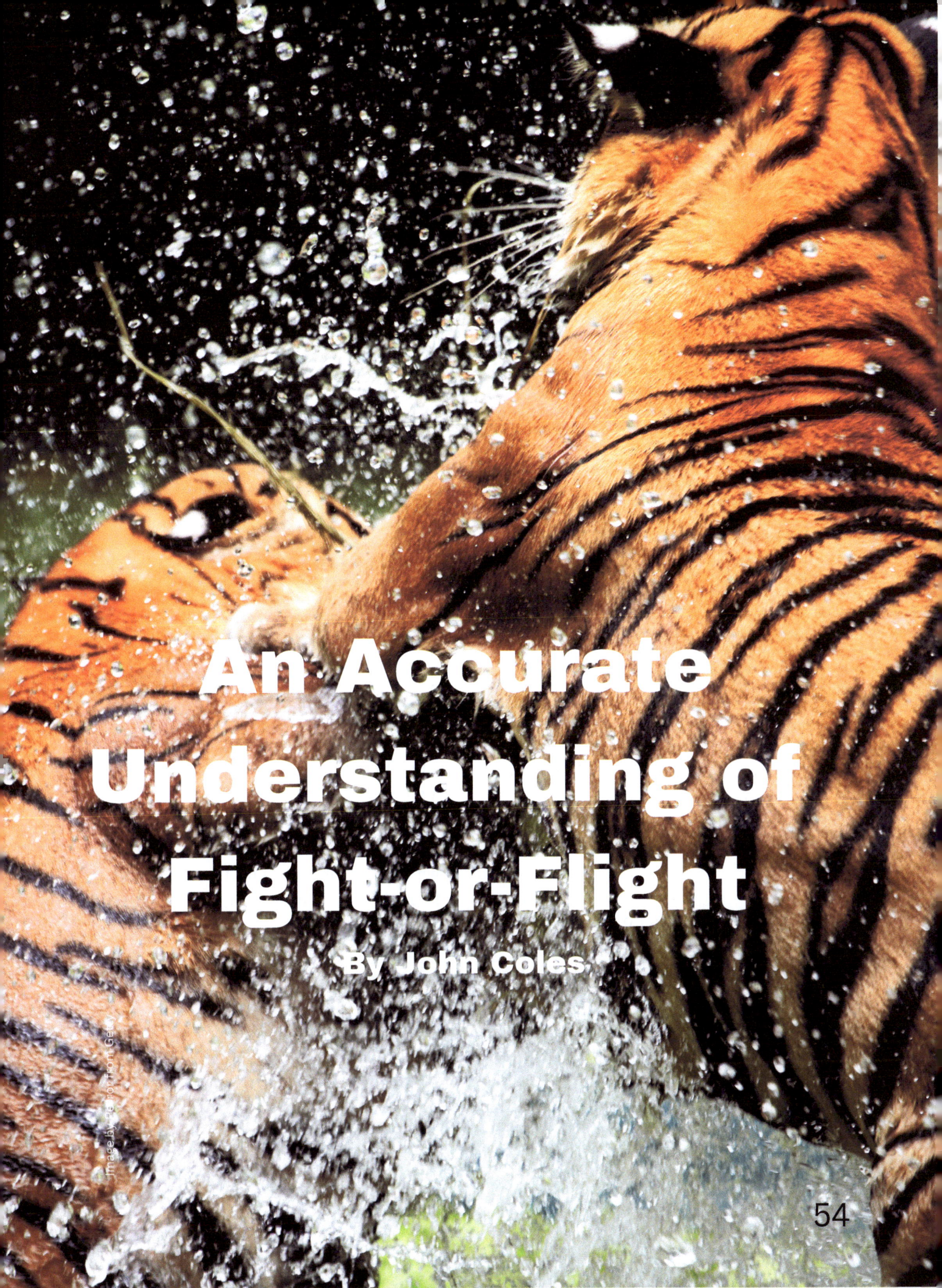

An Accurate Understanding of Fight-or-Flight

By John Coles

This article is adapted from a chapter in my forthcoming book, Fear and Fight: Understanding Our Natural and Learned Responses to a Threat.

Martial arts, self-defence, law enforcement, and military instructors—as well as medical and mental health professionals—frequently invoke the fight-or-flight concept to explain our natural response to a threat. However, this widely accepted framework is often misunderstood, both in its interpretation and in its foundational concept. In this article, I will examine the common misconceptions surrounding fight-or-flight and delve into the limitations of the model itself.

Walter Bradford Cannon and Fight-or-Flight
The term 'fight-or-flight' originates from Walter Bradford Cannon's work in Bodily Changes in Pain, Hunger, Fear and Rage (1915), where he described a survival mechanism designed to protect an individual when their survival is at risk. This mechanism involves physiological, emotional, and behavioural components. Let's briefly examine these components.

Fight-or-Flight Emotional Response(s)

The fight-or-flight concept is commonly associated with fear, yet this is only part of the picture. Walter Cannon, who first described the concept, made a critical distinction between the emotions driving each instinctive behaviour: flight is driven by fear, while fight is fuelled by anger. As Cannon noted, 'the emotion of fear is associated with the instinct for flight, and the emotion of anger or rage with the instinct for fighting or attack' (p. 187).

This distinction is often overlooked, but it is central to understanding fight-or-flight. If fight were an instinctive response to fear, there would be no need to overcome fear to engage in fighting. Instead, the shift from fear to anger is Nature's mechanism for transforming the instinct for flight into the readiness for fight.

Fight-or-Flight Physiological Response

Brown and Fee (2002) describe Cannon as the 'pioneer physiologist of emotion,' noting his early interest in the physiological basis of emotional states. In 1897, Cannon observed that peristaltic waves in the stomach abruptly ceased when his experimental animals were frightened or otherwise disturbed. This observation led to his groundbreaking investigations into the physiology of emotion, making him the first major researcher to systematically study this topic.

Cannon found that emotional states like fear and anger were associated with physiological changes. However, his research in the 1920s concluded that both emotions triggered the same autonomic reactions, leading to the assumption that fear and anger caused identical physiological responses in humans. This view overlooked observable differences, such as changes in facial colouration: fear causes the face to pale as blood is redirected, while anger causes the face to flush as blood flows toward it. Later research confirmed these distinctions, showing that different emotions are accompanied by distinct physiological responses.

Levenson (2003) introduced the concept of autonomic specificity—the idea that emotions can be distinguished by their unique patterns of autonomic nervous system activity. As he put it, 'autonomic specificity is one of those ideas that is just too good not to be true" (p. 214; emphasis in original). Levenson explained that different emotions reliably elicit different behaviours, each requiring specific autonomic configurations.

This hypothesis was supported by earlier work from Levenson, Ekman, and Friesen (1990), who found that anger increased finger temperature, while fear caused a decrease. These findings suggest that fear redirects blood flow toward the torso to support flight, while anger increases blood flow to the hands, preparing for fight-related actions such as grasping or striking.

Fight-or-Flight Behavioural Responses

The fight-or-flight model describes two instinctive responses to a threat: fight and flight. However, the 'or' in fight-or-flight is often misunderstood to suggest an equal choice between these behaviours. Research, particularly in animal studies, indicates that flight is the default response, with fight occurring only when escape is not an option—flee when you can, fight if you must.

Over time, the fight-or-flight model has been criticised for over- is the addition of freeze, which technically refers to tonic immobility—an involuntary, catatonic state often described as being 'frozen with fear' or 'scared stiff.' Bracha et al. (2004) redefined freeze as a 'stop, look, and listen' response, distinguishing it from fright, which they used to describe tonic immobility. This reinterpretation expanded the model into a 4Fs framework: freeze, flight, fight, and fright—occurring sequentially as the threat draws closer.

Bracha (2004) later introduced faint as a fifth response, creating the 5Fs framework. These responses unfold in order: freeze (stop, look, and listen) when the threat is distant; flight as the threat moves closer; fight if escape is obstructed; fright (tonic immobility) as a last resort, signalling submission; and faint, which may serve a similar submissive function while also reducing psychological trauma by blunting memory formation. These revisions highlight the complexity of human threat responses, offering a far more nuanced understanding than the original fight-or-flight model.

It is worth noting that the 5Fs are associated with distinct emotions. The fifth edition of the American Psychiatric Association's Diagnostic and Statistical Manual of Mental Disorders (2013) differentiates fear from anxiety, defining fear as the emotional response to real or perceived imminent threats, while anxiety pertains to the anticipation of future threats. Within this framework, freeze corresponds to anxiety; flight to fear; fight to anger; fright to high-intensity fear or terror and lack of anger; and faint to an absence of emotion.

As I discuss in my forthcoming book, the subjective feeling associated with each response motivates the instinctive behaviour, which the body's physiological reactions prepare to enact.

For example, the first four Fs involve activation of the sympathetic nervous system, mobilising the body for action. In contrast, the fifth F, faint, is characterised by reduced sympathetic nervous system activity and increased parasympathetic nervous system activity, both aimed at aiding survival in specific contexts.

Taylor et al. (2000) proposed an alternative model, tend-and-befriend, to account for behaviours more commonly observed in females under threat. This response involves nurturing actions and seeking social support, shaped by the distinct evolutionary pressures of caregiving. However, females also exhibit the 5F responses, and Taylor et al. acknowledged that males can display tend-and-befriend behaviours as well. Together, these critiques and expansions underscore the multifaceted nature of instinctive threat responses, challenging the simplicity of the original fight-or-flight concept.

Moving Beyond the Fight-or-Flight Concept

While the fight-or-flight concept is limited, we shouldn't discard it altogether. An accurate understanding of fight-or-flight serves as the foundation for a deeper comprehension of our natural responses to threats. This understanding, in turn, informs the methods used by martial arts, self-defence, law enforcement, and military training to help individuals overcome fear and fight when confronted by danger.

One practical application of this understanding is adopting nature's strategy of transforming fear into anger, effectively converting the instinct for flight into the readiness for fight. This approach is especially relevant in self-defence, where emotional control plays a crucial role in overcoming fear. For instance, women's self-defence classes often teach this as a foundational strategy: channelling fear into anger to lower the inhibition to aggress and generate the courage* and strength needed to fight back.

However, this concept is sometimes misunderstood. Some interpretations suggest fear itself can be harnessed directly to fight, a notion rooted in an oversimplification of Cannon's early research, which incorrectly implied identical physiological responses for both fear and anger. In reality, anger uniquely primes the mind and body for confrontation, enabling decisive action in the face of threats.

This strategy is also employed in military contexts. Petersen and Liaras (2006) describe how anger can be strategically used in warfare to counter fear. Historically, warriors have relied on this approach, as seen with the Nordic berserks, who channelled their fear into rage to fight fearlessly. Similarly, Sun Tzu's The Art of War (5th century BC) advises generals to 'arouse the anger of our men' to enhance combat effectiveness (Sun Tzu 1988, p. 108).

By reframing fear as a trigger for anger, these applications underscore the importance of understanding and intentionally directing our emotional responses to threats. For women's self-defence, in particular, this approach not only empowers individuals to overcome fear but also counters misconceptions about how fear physiologically prepares us for action.

While the fight-or-flight concept provides a useful starting point for understanding our responses to threats, it is essential to recognise its limitations. An accurate understanding of the original fight-or-flight mechanism, along with its physiological and emotional components, forms the basis for developing more effective strategies to manage fear and engage in fight when necessary.

Martial arts, self-defence, law enforcement, and military training all rely on interventions that alter the natural response to a threat. Understanding the nuances of how fear, anger, and other emotions shape our behaviour is key to improving these interventions and preparing individuals for life-threatening situations. There is much more to explore in my forthcoming book, but I hope this article provides valuable insight to instructors and practitioners in these fields.

Endnote

In my forthcoming book, I explore the relationship between anger and courage in a chapter on the 'enigma of courage.' As Biswas-Diener explains in Courage Quotient: How Science Can Make You Braver (2012), anger is central to courage:

If fear is the emotion that holds us back from action, then it makes sense that a stronger emotional reaction can overpower that fear and lead us to swift action. In the human palette of feelings there is really only one emotion that is strong enough to overcome fear and that is anger. ... In short, feelings of anger put our bodies on course to act quickly and strongly, often overriding our doubts about our abilities or our concerns with self-preservation. Although anger has something of a bad reputation as a feeling, it is nevertheless the emotion of courage. (p. 59)

By leveraging anger's unique power to overcome fear, this strategy underscores the importance of understanding and directing our emotions effectively, whether in self-defence or broader contexts where courage is required.

References:
American Psychiatric Association 2013, Diagnostic and statistical manual of mental disorders, 5th edn, American Psychiatric Association, Virginia.
Biswas-Diener, R 2012, The courage quotient: How science can make you braver, Jossey-Bass, San Francisco.
Bracha, HS 2004, 'Freeze, flight, fight, fright, faint: Adaptationist perspectives on the acute stress response spectrum', CNS Spectrums, vol. 9, no. 9, pp. 679-685.
Bracha, HS, Ralston, TC, Matsukawa, SM, Williams, AE, & Bracha, AS 2004, 'Does "fight or flight" need updating?', Psychosomatics, vol. 45, no. 5, pp. 448-449.
Brown, TM & Fee, E 2002, 'Walter Bradford Cannon', American Journal of Public Health, vol. 92, no. 10, pp. 1594-1595.
Cannon, WB 1915, Bodily changes in pain, hunger, fear and rage: An account of recent researches into the function of emotional excitement, D. Appleton, New York.
Levenson, RW 2003, 'Autonomic specificity and emotion', in RJ Davidson, KR Scherer, & HH Goldsmith (eds), Handbook of affective sciences, Oxford University Press.
Levenson, RW, Ekman P, & Friesen WV 1990, 'Voluntary facial action generates emotion-specific autonomic nervous system activity', Psychophysiology, vol. 27, no. 4, pp. 363-384.
Petersen, R & Liaras, E 2006, 'Countering fear in war: The strategic use of emotion', Journal of Military Ethics, vol. 5, no. 4, pp. 317-333.
Sun Tzu (5th century BCE) 1988, The art of war, trans. T Cleary, Shambhala, Boston.
Taylor, SE, Klein, LC, Lewis, BP, Gruenewald, TL, Gurung, RAR, & Updegraff, JP 2000, 'Biobehavioral responses to stress in females: Tend-and-befriend, not fight-or-flight', Psychological Review, vol. 107, no. 3, pp. 411-429.

John Coles holds the rank of sandan in jujutsu, shodan in aikido, and third grade in pencak silat under Jan de Jong. He began training in 1983 and started teaching for Jan de Jong in 1985. Coles has taught martial arts in Australia, as well as in Sweden, Denmark, Norway, the Netherlands, Belgium, France, England, Ireland, and Indonesia.

He is the author of Jan de Jong: The Man, His School and His Ju Jitsu System, which has been sold throughout Australia, New Zealand, and Western Europe. In addition, Coles has written numerous articles published in Blitz Australasian Martial Arts and maintains two blogs: Kojutsukan: The Place for the Study of Martial Arts Skills and The School of Jan de Jong.

This article is based on a chapter from his forthcoming book, The Science Behind All Fighting Techniques, which is extensively researched and written by John Coles.

62

An Equation for Excellence
by Kayne M. Dewhurst

Plus, Minus and Equal (PME) is a learning strategy popular with all kinds of leaders. Often attributed to UFC legend Frank Shamrock, the martial arts community has put it to use for decades.

The idea is not complex. In order to become great in your chosen pursuit, you require the assistance of three different people. The first is someone greater from whom you can learn. Next is someone lesser you can teach. The final person is someone similar who can challenge you. These form the Plus, Minus and Equal.

It's not surprising that this concept came from martial arts. Look at your own journey. We stand in line, ordered by grade and learning from the most experienced people in the room. The structure lends itself to finding people who suit your PME system. As you continue to learn and develop, your position in the training landscape changes.

Who are your Plus, Minus or Equal? It may be a single person or a group who fill each of these roles for you. These people are likely clearly defined.

Plus: The "Plus" is someone who is greater or more knowledgeable than you. These people guide your growth, and it is your responsibility to learn. In martial arts, the first person to fill this role is obvious; your instructor. The Japanese teaching title Sensei translates to "one who comes before." Your instructor is further along the same path, and they have already been in your current position. Whether you sought them out or were just lucky enough to stumble into their dojo, they have invested time into your learning. Your instructor even has their own Plus, a coach of their own, and is still growing and learning. Even very established coaches still find opportunities to learn.

"Every man I meet is my master in some point, and in that I learn of him" - Ralph Waldo Emerson

Your Sensei is not the only person who can fill this role. There are others with something to teach. More experienced or more talented, the place you train is filled with people who can show you how to improve. Consider the classes you attend: who has knowledge to share? You might stand at the top of the line but some within your school are your superior in at least one aspect. Perhaps they have better footwork, faster kicks or can execute a kata with greater proficiency. Learn from them.

Kayne M. Dewhurst has been a martial arts practitioner since 1993. Kayne founded the Centre for Karate Excellence in 2006 and the previously popular **OSMAT**: Open Style Martial Arts Tournament in 2015. Holding a 6th Dan in Karate, he is also a Kickboxing Coach. Kayne splits his time between his hometown of Melbourne, Australia and Phnom Penh, Cambodia. Although he occasionally still teaches public classes for karate and MMA, Kayne primarily coaches school owners and professional fighters.

Raising the Bar in Coaching: Leveraging the Power of Focused Drills for long term student development

by Paul Pirie

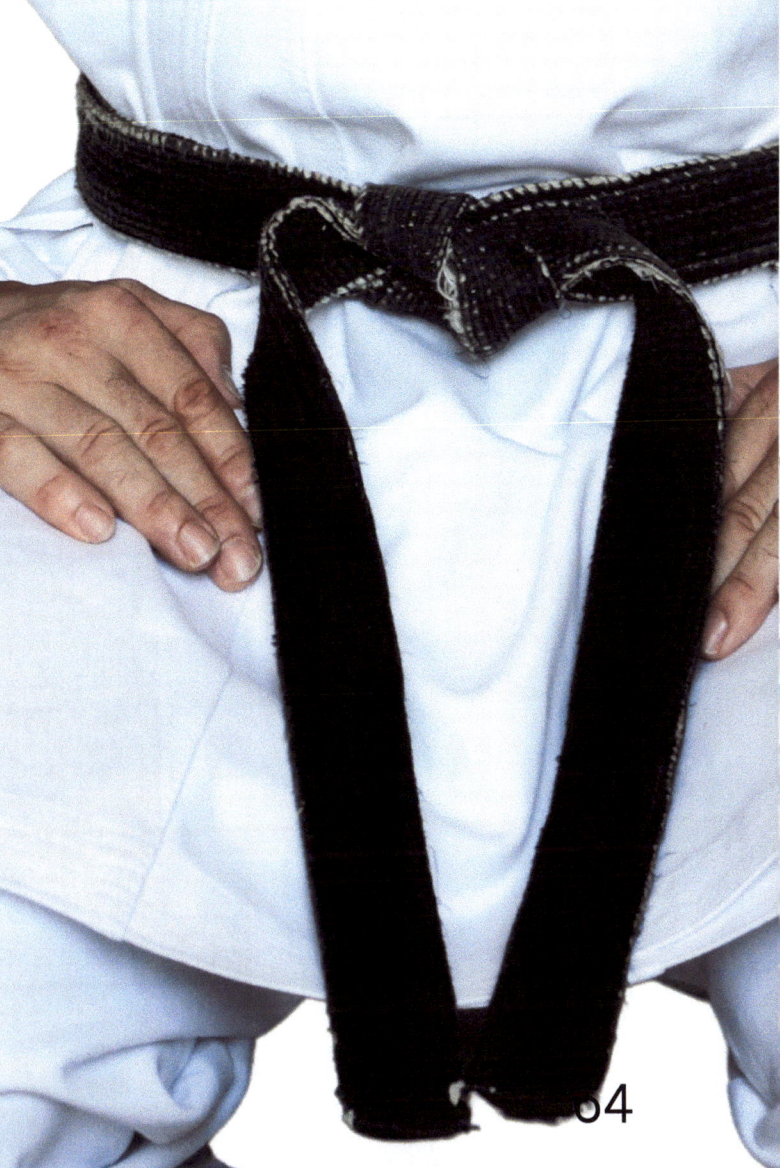

As karate instructors, the challenge is to keep classes both engaging and effective. We've all heard variations of 'something old, something new and something interesting to do' and while it's essential to master specific techniques, avoiding repetitive routines is key to sustaining long-term interest and growth. By refining our approach and targeting various aspects of karate through focused drills, we can help our students build a well-rounded skill set.

Keeping Training Dynamic: The Role of Varied Drills

Variety is crucial in keeping karate training fresh and effective. Rather than simply running through katas, a simple approach for new instructors could be to break them down into their essential components. This approach allows students to deepen their understanding and execution of each movement, ultimately leading to mastery of complex techniques.

For instance, focusing on the finer points of stances, timing, or breath control during a session can significantly enhance a student's overall performance when these elements are later pieced together in kata practice.

The Benefits of a Daily Training Intent

Begin each class with a clear "focus of the class" that targets a specific aspect of your karate technique. For example, if the focus is on breath work, drills might include:

1. Breath Control Exercises - Practising deep, controlled breathing to maintain calmness and focus.
2. Timing Drills - Coordinating breath with movement to maximise efficiency and power.
3. Kata Application - Integrating breath control and timing within a specific kata sequence.

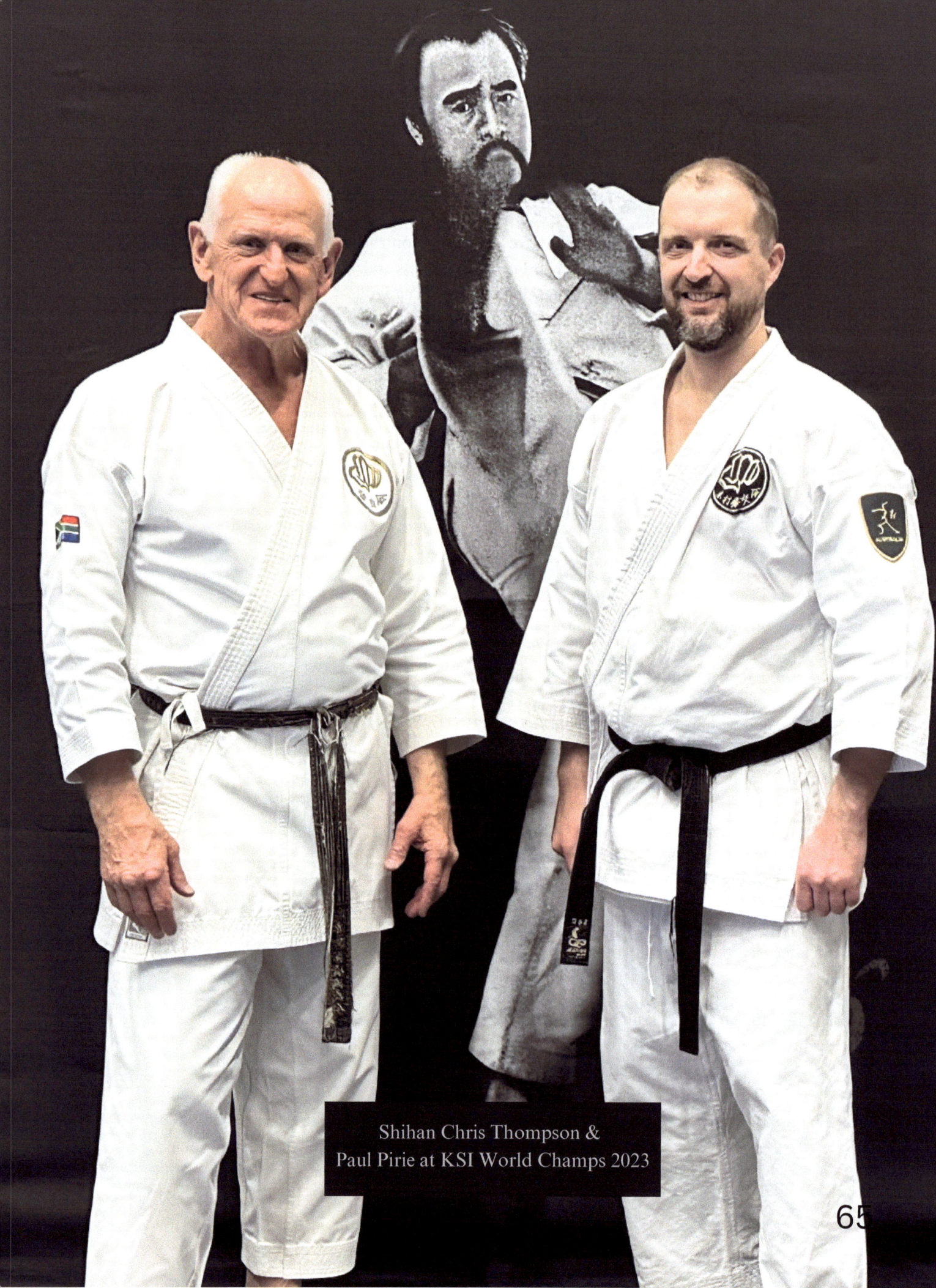

Shihan Chris Thompson & Paul Pirie at KSI World Champs 2023

This approach also ensures that each training session can build on the last, allowing students to internalise key components before progressing to more complex applications.

Learning Through Experimentation and Adaptation

New instructors might find it challenging to structure classes around a specific focus, but this practice is crucial for both personal growth and student development. As you explore different aspects of karate, you'll uncover nuances in techniques that deepen your understanding.

Experimentation is also essential. Trying new drills, even if some don't work as expected, leads to valuable insights and adaptations that can benefit your students. Trust in your experience, and don't be afraid to innovate.

Conclusion: Embracing Focus and Variety in Karate Training

As you plan your training cycles, remember that combining variety with a focused approach is essential to keeping karate training dynamic and effective. By introducing different drills and honing in on specific performance aspects, you'll maintain student engagement and help them achieve their full potential. Continue to learn, adapt, and innovate, guiding your students to new heights in their karate journey.

Author Bio:

Paul Pirie is a 5th Dan Kimura Shukokai Karate and started his karate journey under Shihan Chris Thompson (9th Dan) in South Africa. Paul and his dojo are active members of Kimura Shukokai International (KSI) and he travels overseas at least once a year to train and learn.

Paul has been teaching karate since 1996 and founded Samurai Dojo Australia – Kimura Shukokai Karate in 2014.

Email: hello@samuraidojo.com.au

Website: www.samuraidojo.com.au

Instagram: Paul has been teaching karate since 1996 and founded Samurai Dojo Australia – Kimura Shukokai Karate in 2014.

Facebook: https://www.facebook.com/SamuraiDojoAustralia

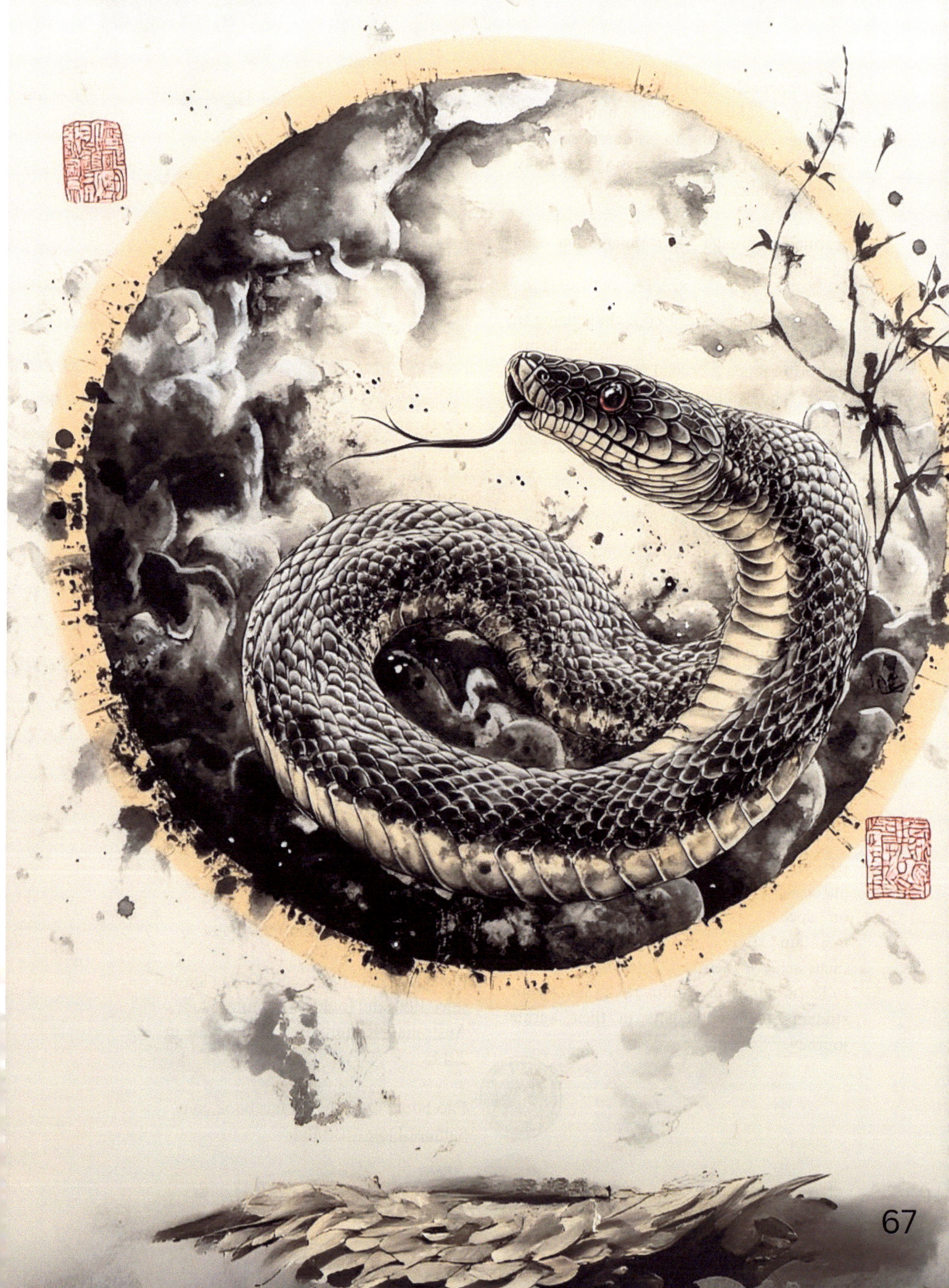

The Enduring Legacy of Jan de Jong: A Personal Journey

by Daniel Newcombe, 6th Dan Tsutsumi Hozan Ryu Jujutsu, 2nd Dan Shotokan Karate

My name is Dan Newcombe, and I am proud to represent the second of three generations in my family to have trained in the jujutsu style taught by Jan de Jong—a tradition believed to be the oldest martial art still practised in Australia today.

Building on Jan de Jong's legacy, I have dedicated myself to expanding his teachings, founding schools in Perth, Western Australia, and contributing to the establishment of a school in the Netherlands. This journey is not just a continuation of Jan de Jong's story—it is also my own.

In this article, I invite you to join me on that journey: to discover how a historic martial art has endured, evolved, and travelled across continents, sustained by the passion and commitment of those who believe in its timeless value.

Jan de Jong's Early Journey

Born in the Dutch East Indies on February 6, 1921, Jan de Jong's martial arts journey began at the age of seven. His introduction to jujutsu came through a fortunate connection facilitated by his father, an engineer, who befriended the Saito brothers in Semarang, Java. Though the Saito brothers were notoriously selective in choosing their students—rarely admitting non-Japanese—de Jong's father's relationship with them granted him access to their dojo.

For over a decade, de Jong trained with the Saito brothers, steadily progressing through the ranks. Little is known about the brothers, even by de Jong himself, as they were highly private individuals, rarely speaking about their personal lives. By the time he left for Holland in 1939 to pursue his dream of becoming a pilot, he had achieved his third dan—a remarkable accomplishment. At just 18 years old, he had reached the highest technical grade in the system, though higher ranks were reserved for those older than him. Still, his commitment and skill were evident, setting the stage for the remarkable martial artist he would become.

Resilience Amidst War

In this article, I invite you to join me on that journey: to discover how a historic martial art has endured, evolved, and travelled across continents, sustained by the passion and commitment of those who believe in its timeless value.

De Jong's plans were abruptly disrupted in 1940 when the Nazis invaded Holland. In the face of war, he opened his first jujutsu school in Rotterdam, growing it to 300 students despite the constant threat of forced labour roundups by the German occupiers. De Jong cleverly avoided conscription by forging university documents, and he also joined the Dutch Resistance, risking his life to fight the occupying forces.

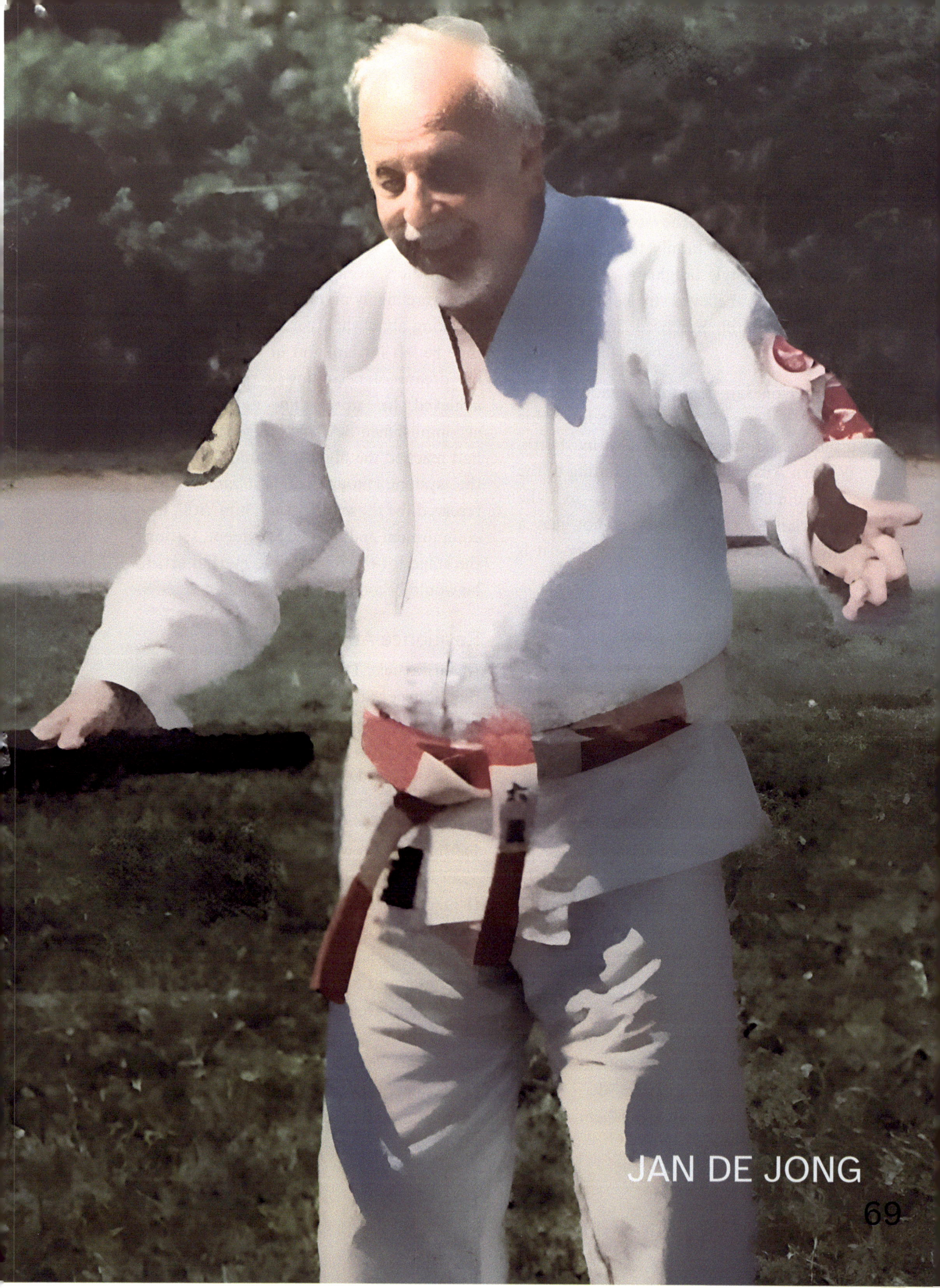

JAN DE JONG

After the war, de Jong trained as a physiotherapist and, in 1946, returned to Indonesia. During this time, which coincided with the War of Independence following WWII, he accepted a civilian position as a physiotherapist with the Royal Netherlands Indies Army (KNIL). While in Indonesia, de Jong also began training in the indigenous martial art of pencak silat under Guru Soehadi of the Suci Hati aliran. By 1951, he had attained the equivalent of a sixth-degree black belt in silat, further deepening his martial arts expertise.

A New Beginning in Australia

In 1952, after a decade spent in war zones —five years in Europe during WWII and five years in Indonesia amidst the war of independence—de Jong emigrated to Perth, Western Australia, seeking stability and a warmer climate. His time in both Europe and Indonesia had been fraught with conflict, including an unsettling experience where his family was held at gunpoint during a home invasion by Indonesian freedom fighters. This period of turmoil undoubtedly influenced his decision to start anew in Australia.

Initially working as a labourer, de Jong began teaching martial arts during lunch breaks. By 1963, he had established himself as Australia's first full-time martial arts instructor. Reflecting on this era in the foreword to the book Jan de Jong: The Man, His School and His Ju Jitsu System (Coles, 1997), de Jong wrote:

Looking back at my own early years in Australia (1952-1963), self-defence was often considered a rather peculiar and odd thing to do. The term 'judo' was known by some, but most people had not even heard of 'karate' or 'kung fu,' let alone 'ju jitsu.' My expressed intention to make the teaching of this art into my living was almost always met with doubt, if not ridicule. The idea that anyone could teach an oriental self-defence professionally was not considered possible. However, I had the confidence that I could and would do this. When I did make it my full-time occupation in 1963, to the best of my knowledge, I was the only full-time martial arts instructor in Australia.

In 1963, de Jong established a permanent dojo on the edge of Perth's CBD, a spacious facility featuring four large mat areas. Two years later, in 1965, he opened his first suburban branch, paving the way for the establishment of numerous additional branches across Perth's suburban areas in the following years. Under his leadership, the school flourished, eventually enrolling over 1,000 students—a remarkable achievement, particularly considering Perth's relatively small population at the time.

In 1968, de Jong was introduced to Yoseikan aikido by Philippe Boiron, a student of Minoru Mochizuki. This inspired De Jong to travel to Japan in 1969, at the age of 48, where he trained directly under Mochizuki as a live-in student (uchideshi). Upon returning to Australia, De Jong began teaching aikido, and in 1974, he sponsored Yoshiaki Unno, a highly credentialed martial artist from Mochizuki's school, to teach aikido and karate at his school. De Jong and his son, Hans, trained intensively with Unno for two years, six days a week.

Over the years, de Jong and his instructors also taught self-defence in numerous high schools and for various organisations. Of particular note was his collaboration with Major Greg Mawkes MBE (retired), who secured de Jong's expertise to modernise the Australian Army's unarmed combat training. Reflecting on this partnership, Mawkes observed:

Since 1978, I have conducted unarmed combat courses for both the SAS and the Commandos. It is my sincere hope that the young men I have trained never find it necessary to use their skills but if they do, I am confident that they will be extremely effective. If what they know helps save their lives, then it is Jan de Jong to whom they should be grateful. (Coles 1997, p. 23)

National and International Recognition

In 1978, despite having vowed never to return to Europe after experiencing the Dutch famine of 1944-1945 (known as the Hunger Winter), where 22,000 people perished from severe winter and lack of food supplies, de Jong returned to Europe to assess the jujutsu scene. This marked the beginning of a new phase in his career. Following his initial visit, de Jong received numerous invitations to conduct seminars across Europe. In 1982, he returned with a team of instructors for what became an annual tour. Over the next two decades, he would conduct seminars in Austria, Belgium, Denmark, England, France, Germany, Holland, Indonesia, Italy, Malaysia, New Zealand, Norway, Poland, Spain, Sweden, the United States of America, and throughout Australia.

As a consequence of his increasing international reputation, students and instructors from around Australia and Europe would travel to Perth to train with de Jong and his instructors. His expertise gained international acclaim. In the 1980s, de Jong became the Australian representative for the World Ju Jitsu Federation (WJJF) and the International Pencak Silat Federation. This was followed by his appointment as President and National Coach for the Australian Ju Jitsu Association (AJJA) in 1987, and

Vice President of the WJJF in 1989. While these were political positions, de Jong remained focused on improving techniques and strengthening both jujutsu itself and the image it held. Brierley Baily OAM, National Secretary of the AJJA, credits de Jong's presence within the AJJA with bringing jujutsu together around Australia and advancing it on the world stage. His achievements were officially recognised by the Australian Government when he was awarded the Order of Australia Medal in 1990 for services to the martial arts in Australia.

Jan de Jong passed away on April 5, 2003, leaving behind a profound legacy. His teachings continue to thrive locally, nationally, and internationally. In Perth and surrounding areas, at least ten schools trace their origins to the original Jan de Jong Self Defence School continuing to teach his jujutsu — 'like streams endlessly dividing as they flow outward from their original source' (Friday 1997, p. 18). Across Australia, several other schools credit their teachings to Jan de Jong, as do a number of schools in Western Europe.

Tsutsumi Hozan Ryu

Jan de Jong credited his instructors in Indonesia with teaching him the jujutsu style known as Tsutsumi Hozan Ryu (THR). This tradition became the cornerstone of de Jong's teachings, shaping the unique system he shared in Australia and, eventually, worldwide. Although the precise origins and details of this style remain somewhat elusive, THR holds a central place in the martial arts philosophy that de Jong championed throughout his career.

Over nearly 40 years of involvement in the de Jong jujutsu tradition, I have developed an enduring fascination with the history behind this art. My fascination began, when I wrote a black belt (shodan) history essay on the subject. This essay was part of the innovative grading system introduced by de Jong, designed to produce not only skilled practitioners but also high-quality instructors. While de Jong envisioned separate streams for practitioners and instructors, he did not live to fully implement this concept. Inspired by his vision, I later developed these dual pathways within my own branch of the Jan de Jong tradition, ensuring that both streams honour his legacy.

Over the past five years, I have conducted extensive research into the history of THR, accessing Japanese source materials and resources that were unavailable to Western audiences even a few years ago. My work has uncovered a wealth of information that connects the origins of THR in fourteenth-century Japan to the version taught by Jan de Jong.

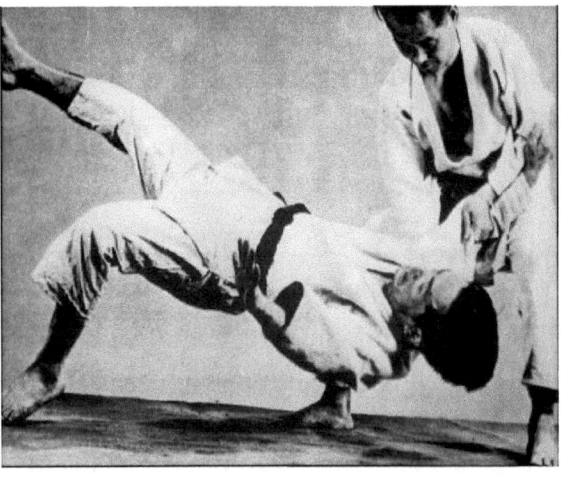

Saito Brothers - Jan de Jongs Sensei circa 1930

This research also informed my teaching at the schools I founded in Perth, as well as the organisation and grading system I co-founded in the Netherlands with Wim Mallens, —marking a significant step in expanding de Jong's legacy to Western Europe. De Jong is also known to have loved teaching in Europe and his teaching was much sought after however he did not take the next step in establishing a school there, although he often expressed an interest in doing so. Wim Mallens and I have effectively realised this ambition by reintroducing the system to the Netherlands, where it was last taught in the 1940s, integrating it into his successful school, Tadashii-Do. Together, we aim to ensure that this timeless art continues to thrive.

The findings of my research will culminate in a forthcoming book, which will trace the evolution of THR from its historical roots to its modern practice within the Jan de Jong tradition.

In a follow-up article, I will provide a brief summary of the findings of my research into the THR tradition. This will include some fascinating insights that challenge certain widely accepted doctrines associated with jujutsu and Kodokan Judo.

References
Friday, KF 1997, Legacies of the sword: The Kashima-Shinryu and samurai martial culture, University of Hawai'i Press, Honolulu.
Coles, J 1997, Jan de Jong: The man, his school and his ju jitsu system, Jan de Jong Self Defence School, Perth, Western Australia.

Author
Dan Newcombe has been a a practicing engineer for 30 years and an active practitioner and teacher of jujutsu from the de Jong tradition in Perth, Western Australia for close to 40 years. Dan started his training with the Jan de Jong Self Defence School in 1986, and continued his training with the Hans De Jong Self Defence School after de Jong passed away in 2003. Dan founded self defence schools teaching the de Jong lineage jujutsu in Perth from 2010 and is now primarily occupied with conducting workshops, personal training, assessments and standardisation of related gradings in the Netherlands and Perth for associated clubs.

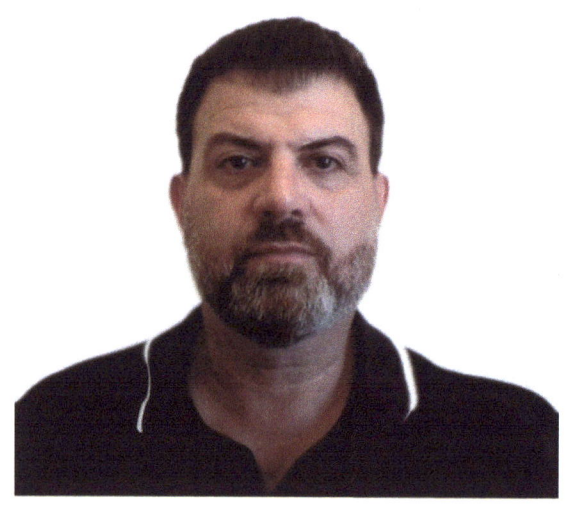

Daniel Newcombe, 6th Dan Tsutsumi Hozan Ryu Jujutsu, 2nd Dan Shotokan Karate.
Founder of Colosseum Martial Arts and Self Defence Central Dojo.
Co-Founder and Principal of Tsutsumi Hozan Ryu International, an organisation established to support client schools by providing a standardised grading system, along with accredited instructors and examiners.

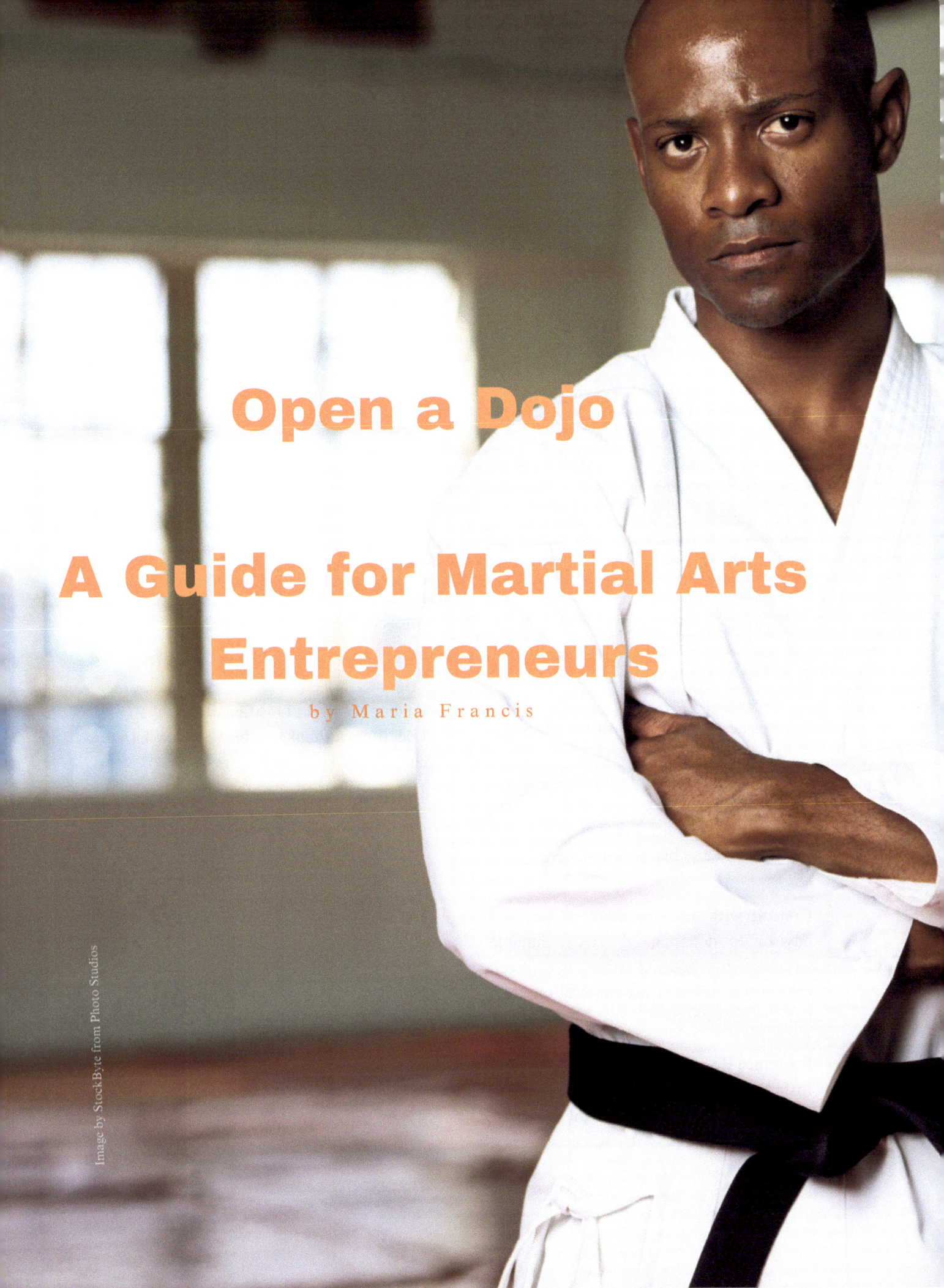

Open a Dojo

A Guide for Martial Arts Entrepreneurs

by Maria Francis

In the ever expanding landscape of martial arts instruction in Australia, opening a karate club represents both an exciting opportunity and a significant challenge. Whether you're a seasoned instructor looking to branch out on your own or an experienced practitioner ready to share your knowledge, establishing a successful dojo requires careful planning, understanding of legal requirements, and a solid business strategy.

Business Registration and Structure
The first step in establishing your karate club is deciding on your business structure. Most new dojos start as sole proprietorships or partnerships, though some opt for a company structure for additional protection and scalability.

In Australia you will need:
- An Australian Business Number (ABN): Apply through the Australian Business Register
- Business name registration: Register through ASIC Connect
- Tax File Number (TFN): Essential for tax reporting
- Business bank account: Separate personal and business finances

Consult with an accountant or business advisor to determine the most suitable structure for your circumstances. Each option has different tax implications and liability considerations.

Insurance Requirements
Insurance is non-negotiable when operating a martial arts club. Essential coverage includes:

1. Public Liability Insurance
   - Minimum cover of $10 - 20 million
   - Protects against third party injury
   - Coverage for property damage

2. Professional Indemnity Insurance
   - Covers advice related claims
   - Typically $5 - 10 million coverage

3. Building and Contents Insurance
   - Coverage for equipment and facilities
   - Protection against theft or damage
   - Business interruption coverage

Many insurance providers offer specialised martial arts instruction packages. Check that you are covered for everything that need and that you are not paying for policies that look good on paper but have little substance in protecting you and your students.

Finding the Right Location
Location can make or break a new karate club. Consider these factors:

1. Accessibility
   - Proximity to public transport
   - Adequate parking
   - Visibility from main roads
   - Local demographic match

2. Space Requirements
   - Min 100 -150 sq m for small classes
   - High ceilings for high kicks and jumping techniques
   - Adequate ventilation
   - Change room facilities
   - Storage space for equipment

3. Lease Considerations
- Length of lease term
- Rent increases and reviews
- Maintenance responsibilities
- Fit out allowances
- Council approval requirements

Many successful dojos start in shared or temporary spaces:

1. Community Centres
- Lower initial costs
- Flexible booking options
- Established facilities
- Built in community presence

2. School Halls
- Available after hours
- Suitable floor space
- Cost effective starting point
- Potential student base nearby

3. Existing Gyms
- Shared facility arrangements
- Ready made amenities
- Potential cross promotion
- Reduced overhead costs

Essential Equipment
Initial equipment investment should include:

1. Training Surfaces
- Martial arts mats
- Impact absorption rating suitable for throws
- Easy cleaning and maintenance

2. Safety Equipment
- First aid kits
- Crash mats
- Training pads and shields
- Emergency contact information

3. Teaching Tools
- Mirrors for technique correction
- Timer/clock
- Whistles/bells
- Documentation storage

4. Student Equipment
- Basic protective gear for loan
- Training weapons if required
- Spare uniforms for new students

Timetable Development
Creating an effective class schedule requires balancing several factors:

1. Peak Times
- After school/work hours
- Saturday mornings
- Early morning adult classes

2. Age Group Considerations
- Children's classes
- Teen classes
- Adult beginners and advanced
- Family classes

3. Specialty Programs
- Competition training
- Self-defence workshops
- Corporate programs
- School holiday programs

Class Format

Structured classes help maintain quality and consistency:

1. Standard Class Structure
   - Warm up (10 - 15 mins)
   - Technical training (20 - 30 mins)
   - Application practice (15 - 20 mins)
   - Cool down and review (5 -10 mins)

2. Progression System
   - Clear grading requirements
   - Regular assessment opportunities
   - Achievement recognition
   - Documented syllabus

Digital Presence

Establish a strong online presence with:

1. Website
   - Professional design
   - Clear class information
   - Online booking system
   - Blog/content section

2. Social Media
   - Regular content posting
   - Student success stories
   - Training tips and insights
   - Community engagement

3. Google Business Profile
   - Location and hours
   - Photos and videos
   - Student reviews
   - Regular updates

Local Marketing

Community based marketing:

1. School Programs
   - After school activities
   - Physical education demonstrations
   - Holiday programs
   - School newsletter advertising

2. Community Events
   - Local festivals
   - Shopping center demonstrations
   - Community group presentations
   - Charity events

3. Referral Programs
   - Student incentives
   - Family discounts
   - Friend trial classes
   - Cross promotion

Pricing Strategy

Develop a sustainable pricing structure:

1. Membership Options
   - Casual rates
   - Term payments
   - Annual memberships
   - Family packages

2. Additional Revenue Streams
   - Private lessons
   - Seminars and workshops
   - Equipment sales
   - Grading fees

3. Payment Systems
   - Direct debit arrangements
   - Point of sale system
   - Online payment options
   - Record keeping software

Cost Management
Control expenses with careful planning:

1. Fixed Costs
   Rent/venue hire
   Insurance
   Utilities
   Marketing budget

2. Variable Costs
   Equipment replacement
   Cleaning supplies
   Training materials

Instructor Qualifications
Maintain and upgrade professional standards:

1. Required Certifications
   - First Aid and CPR
   - Working with Children Check
   - Style specific rankings

2. Additional Training
   - Teaching methodology
   - Child protection
   - Risk management
   - Business management

Safety and Compliance
Implement safety protocols:

1. Risk Management
   - Written safety procedures
   - Incident reporting system
   - Emergency action plans
   - Regular equipment checks

2. Student Management
   - Health screening
   - Injury prevention
   - Progress monitoring
   - Behaviour management

Building Community and Retention
Student Engagement
Create a supportive dojo environment:

1. Community Building
   - Social events
   - Training camps
   - Online community groups

2. Parent Involvement
   - Regular communication
   - Progress reports
   - Parent committees
   - Family events

3. Recognition Programs
   - Student of the month
   - Achievement boards
   - Social media highlights
   - Newsletter features

Professional Network
Develop industry relationships:

1. Martial Arts Organizations
   - Style associations
   - Industry bodies
   - Competition circuits
   - Insurance groups

2. Business Networks
   - Local business groups
   - Sports associations
   - Education providers
   - Health professionals

Measuring Success
Monitor key performance indicators:

1. Financial Metrics
   Student numbers

- Revenue per student
- Retention rates
- Profit margins

2. Quality Metrics
- Student progress
- Competition results
- Parent feedback
- Community impact

Planning for Growth
Prepare for future development:

1. Expansion Options
- Additional locations
- Program diversification
- Online training
- Instructor development

2. Business Evolution
- Franchise potential
- Partnership opportunities
- Brand development
- Market positioning

Opening a karate club requires careful planning and execution across multiple areas. Success depends on balancing traditional martial arts values with modern business practices. By focusing on quality instruction, professional management, and community building, new club owners can create sustainable and rewarding businesses that contribute to both the martial arts community and their local area.

The most successful dojos grow organically, building strong foundations before expanding. Take time to develop your systems, nurture your student base, and create a positive training environment. With dedication, proper planning, and attention to detail, your karate club can become a valued part of your community and a successful business venture.

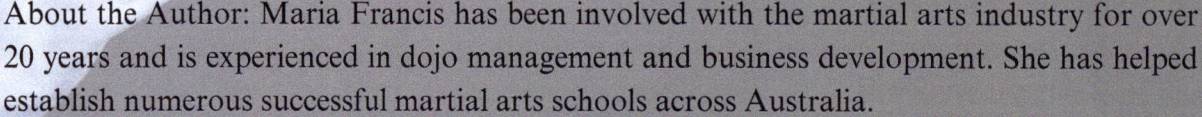
Image by Gyro Getty Images

About the Author: Maria Francis has been involved with the martial arts industry for over 20 years and is experienced in dojo management and business development. She has helped establish numerous successful martial arts schools across Australia.

PINÁN KATA

Foundational Building Blocks of Modern Karate Training

by Don McKay

In the world of traditional karate, few training sequences have shaped the development of practitioners quite like the Pinán kata series. These five fundamental forms, developed by Okinawan master Ankō Itosu in the early 1900s, revolutionised how karate was taught and continue to serve as cornerstone training methods in dojos worldwide.

The creation of the Pinán kata marked a pivotal moment in karate's transition from a secretive martial art to a standardised educational system. Ankō Itosu, recognising the need for a more structured approach to teaching, ingeniously distilled complex movements from advanced kata—particularly the renowned Kusanku (Kanku Dai)—into more digestible sequences.

The name "Pinán" (平安), meaning "peaceful mind" in Okinawan, reflects the kata's intended purpose: to provide students with a clear, systematic path to mastering karate's fundamental principles. In other karate styles, these same forms are known as "Heian," the Japanese pronunciation of the same characters.

The Pinán series consists of five progressive kata:

- Pinán Shodan introduces basic stances and blocking techniques, establishing a strong foundation in fundamental movements.

- Pinán Nidan builds upon basic techniques while introducing more complex combinations and transitional movements.

- Pinán Sandan emphasises quick directional changes and introduces more advanced striking techniques, challenging students to maintain proper form during rapid transitions.

- Pinán Yondan brings in more sophisticated defensive manoeuvres and combination techniques, often incorporating movements that simulate responses to multiple attackers.

- Pinán Godan, the final form, integrates advanced techniques and concepts from the previous kata while introducing unique movements that prepare students for higher level training.

Today, the Pinán kata serve multiple crucial functions in karate training. At the most basic level, they provide a structured curriculum for developing proper technique, stance, and body mechanics. Each kata builds upon the previous ones, creating a comprehensive system for physical development and technical proficiency.

Beyond mere physical technique, these forms teach essential concepts of timing, distance, and angle of attack. Through regular practice, students develop a deeper understanding of martial principles such as economy of movement, power generation, and strategic positioning.

The Pinán series also serves as a bridge between basic training and advanced application. While the movements may appear simple, they contain layers of sophisticated applications (bunkai) that reveal themselves as practitioners advance in their training. This makes the Pinán kata valuable not just for beginners, but for advanced students who continue to discover new depths in these seemingly simple forms.

The genius of Itosu's Pinán system lies in its adaptability. These katas are practiced across numerous karate styles, including Shotokan, Wado ryu, Shito ryu, and various Shorin ryu schools. While the specific details may vary between styles, the core principles remain consistent.

In modern dojos, the Pinán kata continue to fulfill their original purpose: providing a systematic method for developing strong fundamental skills while preparing students for more advanced training. Their endurance as training tools speaks to both their effectiveness and the wisdom of their design.

As karate continues to evolve in the 21st century, the Pinán katas remain relevant, offering practitioners a time-tested method for developing physical technique, mental discipline, and martial understanding. They stand as a testament to the importance of systematic training and the enduring value of traditional teaching methods in modern martial arts practice.

Whether practicing for self-defence, competition, or personal development, students of karate continue to find value in these century old forms, proving that Anko Itosu's innovative teaching method remains as relevant today as when it was first developed.

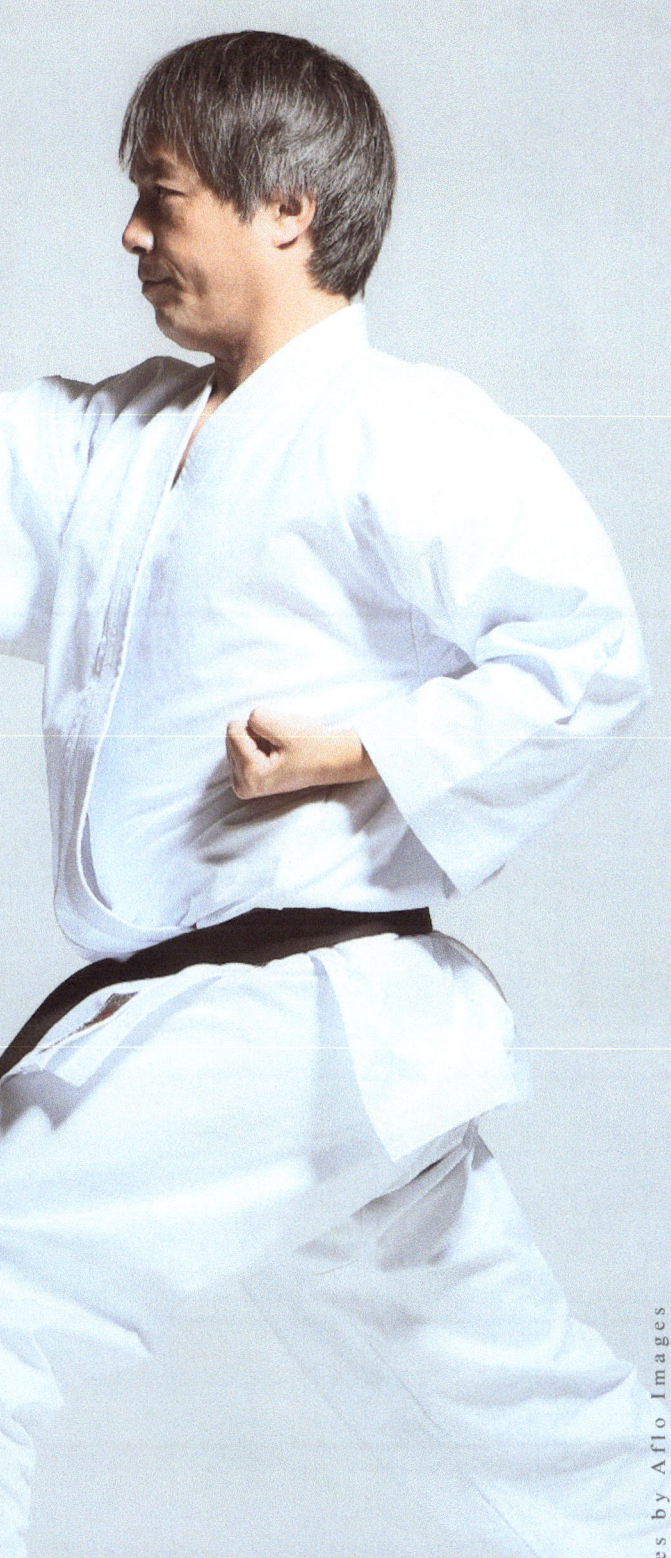

Images by Aflo Images

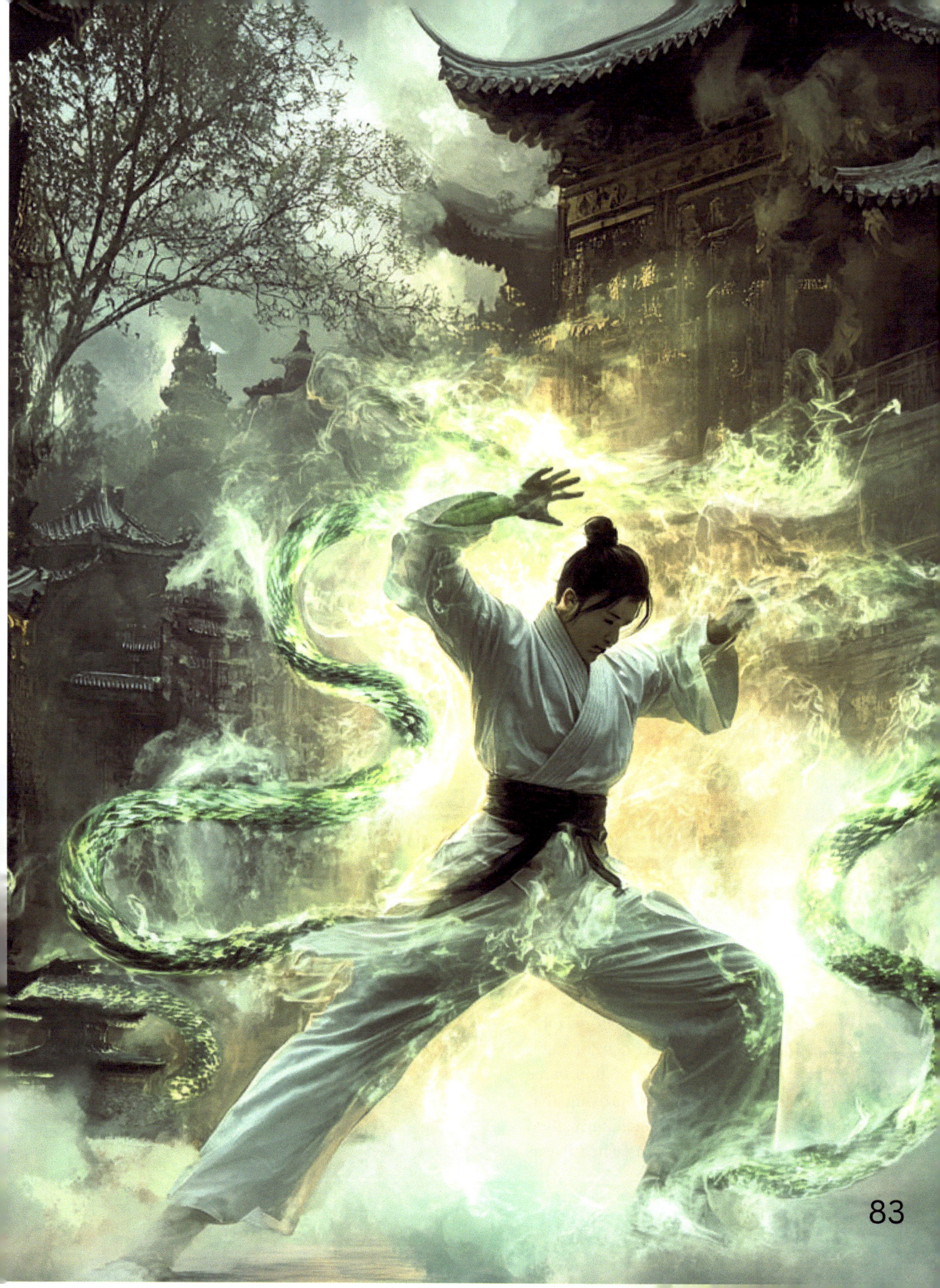

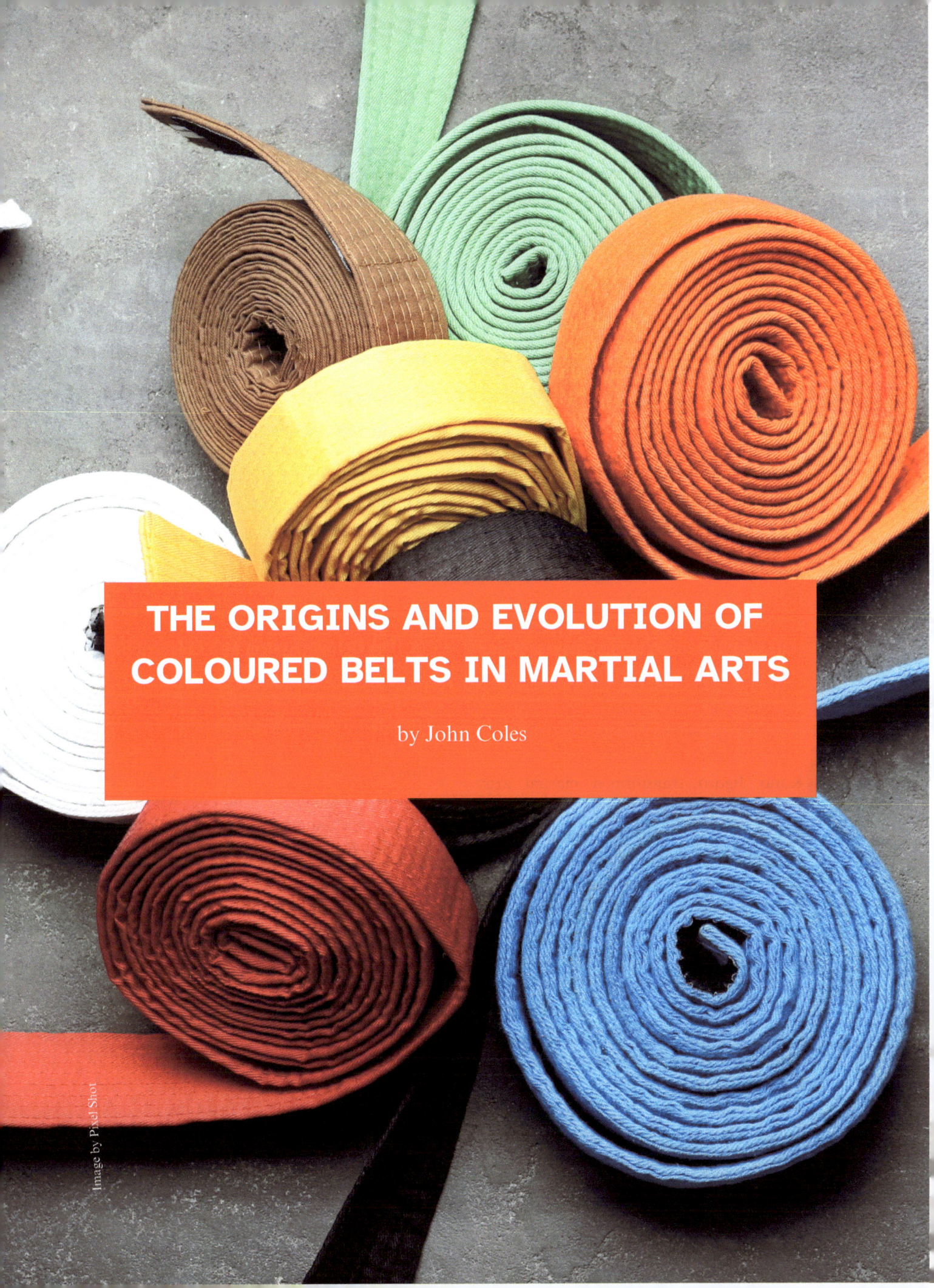

THE ORIGINS AND EVOLUTION OF COLOURED BELTS IN MARTIAL ARTS

by John Coles

The coloured belts seen in martial arts today serve as markers of a practitioner's progression and skill. However, the history of this ranking system is rich and complex, with roots spanning centuries and continents.

Early Beginnings: Diplomas and Licences

The first known martial arts ranking systems emerged in sixteenth-century Japan, where bugei ryuha (martial arts schools) issued certificates to students upon mastery of specific teachings (the menkyo system). Historian Karl Friday (1997), a menkyo kaiden (master license) holder in Kashima Shinryu, suggests that these early diplomas were foundational to formal martial arts rankings. Eventually, disciplines like karate and judo adopted a more standardised system of ranks, symbolised today by coloured belts—a shift largely credited to judo pioneer Kano Jigoro in the late nineteenth century.

Kano Jigoro and the Dan-Kyu System

Kano Jigoro transformed martial arts ranking with the dan-kyu system, introducing a structured approach to indicate a student's skill level. In 1883, Kano awarded the first dan ranks (black belts) to two students, Shiro Saigo and Tomita Tsunejiro, drawing inspiration, as it is said, from Japan's traditional dan system used in Go, a strategy board game, and a swimming ranking system where advanced swimmers wore a black ribbon. Black belts indicated yudansha (black belt holders), while beginners (mudansha) wore white belts. This visible ranking system allowed for easier skill assessment and has since influenced martial arts worldwide.

The Spread of Coloured Belts in Europe

Coloured belts for kyu (below black belt) ranks are often attributed to Mikinosuke Kawaishi, who introduced the system in France in the 1930s. However, records from London's Budokwai judo club—founded in 1918—show that coloured belts were used as early as 1926. Committee notes from 1927 list ranks by colour: white, yellow, green, blue, brown, and black (Callan 2015). This pre-dated Kawaishi's 1928 visit to Budokwai, possibly influencing his system in France. According to the International Judo Federation (2007), the British coloured belt system, established by Gunji Koizumi, may have even been inspired by billiard balls, although the origins are unclear.

A 1906 German System with Coloured Belts

Intriguingly, a coloured belt system predates these developments. In 1906, Masao Tsutsumi and Katsukuma Higashi's book Jiu-Jitsu die große Kunst der Selbstverteidigung und vollendeten Körperausbildung (Jiu-Jitsu: The Great Art of Self-Defence and Complete Physical Training) presented a system with seven coloured belts:

- Red for beginners
- Yellow for sixth rank
- White for fifth rank
- Green for fourth rank
- Orange for third rank
- Purple for second rank
- Black-and-white for first rank

This system precedes known judo ranking methods, raising questions about its origins and influence.

The Cultural Significance of Purple and Black-and-White Belts

Purple has a longstanding association with royalty in Japan, dating back to the Nara period (710–794), when the kan'i jūnikai (twelve-level cap and rank system) designated purple for the highest ranks, reserved for those closest to the emperor. This historical connection to nobility may explain why purple appears as a high-ranking colour in the 1906 German belt system. Additionally, the black-and-white belt in this system symbolises high-level proficiency and remains a rare marker among practitioners, further underscoring its unique status.

Miarka, Marques, and Franchini (2011) note that women's judo black belts often feature a white stripe, symbolising 'purity.' This mirrors the 1906 system's use of a black-and-white belt to denote advanced skill. The authors recount the story of Sarah Meyers, a British female judoka who trained in Japan in the mid-1930s and became the first foreign woman awarded a dan rank in 1935. In a photograph, Meyers is seen wearing a black belt without a white stripe, which the authors suggest reflects her training's equivalence with male standards: 'The belt she wears has no white stripe... no doubt indicating her training was recognised as equivalent to men's' (p. 1023).

These historical and cultural details inspire further questions about the origins and significance of coloured belt systems across martial arts, hinting at a deep-rooted symbolism that has evolved yet still resonates in traditions today.

Personal Reflections on the Evolution of Coloured Belts

The evolution of coloured belts in martial arts is not only an academic history but also one that continues to shape personal experiences within the martial arts community. My own journey with the coloured belt system has highlighted this continuity and complexity. In particular, I trained under Jan de Jong, who implemented a coloured belt ranking system rooted in the German 1906 system described by Tsutsumi and Higashi. This system, with its unique combination of colours and ranks, was the only one I knew—its black-and-white belt for first kyu, or pre-black-belt proficiency, marked a significant milestone.

However, it wasn't until I attended a jujutsu conference in Germany in the 1980s that I discovered just how unique this grading symbol was. Wearing the black-and-white belt, I found myself frequently asked about its meaning by other practitioners, many of whom had never seen such a belt and were curious about its origins. Their questions underscored how distinct this symbol was within the broader martial arts community.

This experience illuminated the often-overlooked diversity within martial arts ranking systems and underscored how these systems can vary by region and lineage. For example, in Japanese tradition, purple has long been associated with high rank, yet in our lineage, the black-and-white belt had come to signify a comparable level of proficiency. These differences invite deeper questions about the cultural and contextual layers embedded in martial arts ranking systems and how traditions like these adapt as they cross borders and are integrated into different martial arts schools worldwide.

Questions and Implications

The existence of a coloured belt system as early as 1906 challenges traditional narratives around martial arts ranking. Why was this German system not referenced in later developments of the dan-kyu system by researchers? Did Kano's judo system evolve independently, or was it influenced by this German system? These questions underscore the layers of cultural and historical significance embedded in martial arts ranking—a system that continues to evolve while respecting its complex origins.

References:

Callen, M 2015, 'History of the grading system', Conference: British Judo Association Senior Examiners, University of Wolverhampton, accessed 12 November 2024, https://www.researchgate.net/publication/299604160_History_of_the_Grading_System

Friday, K 1997, Legacies of the sword: The Kashima-Shinryu and samurai martial culture, University of Hawai'i Press.

International Judo Federation 2007, 'The Belt: Myth and Reality of an Essential Symbol', accessed 12 November 2024, https://www.ijf.org/history/judo-culture/2250

Miarka, B, Marques, JB, and Franchini, E 2011, 'Reinterpreting the history of women's judo in Japan', International Journal of the History of Sport, pp. 1016-1029.

Tsutsumi, M and Higashi K 1906, Jiu-Jitsu die große Kunst der Selbstverteidigung und vollendeten Körperausbildung, Independent, Berlin.

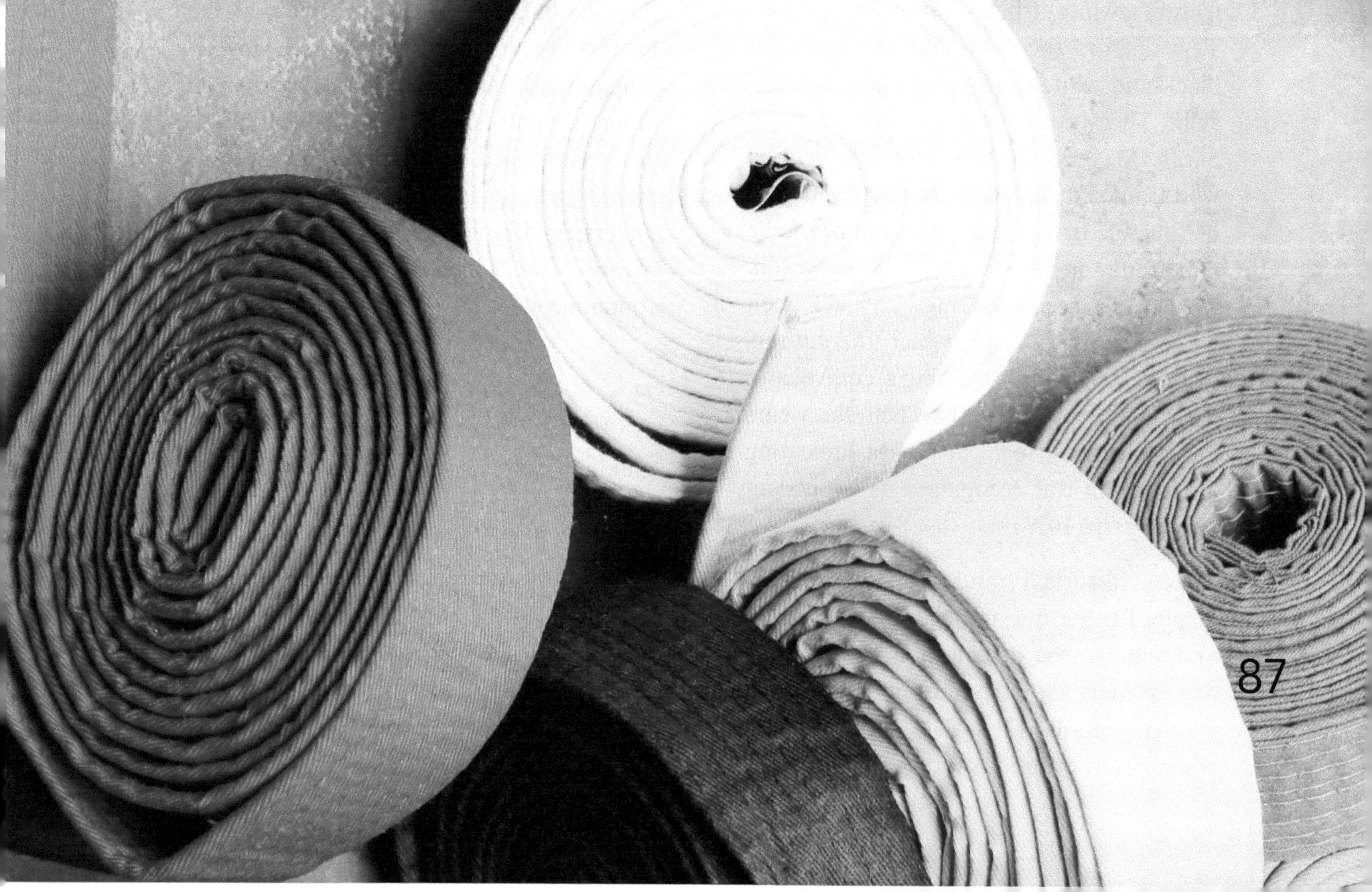

Chicken & Garlic Stir Fry

From Marty's Kitchen

GINGER-GARLIC CHICKEN STIR FRY

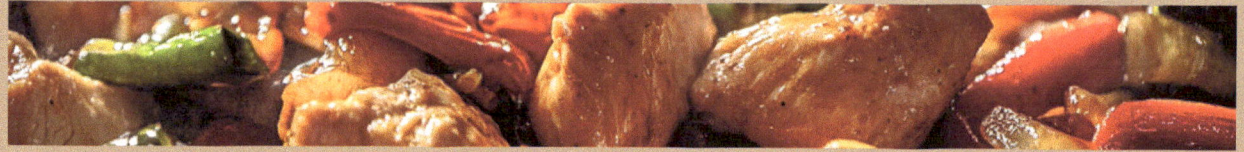

INGREDIENTS

500g chicken breast, cubed
2 tbsp minced ginger
4 garlic cloves
2 cups broccoli
1 bell pepper
2 medium carrots

Sauce: 45ml soy, 15ml rice vinegar, 5ml honey

Garnish: sesame seeds, green onions

METHOD

1. Marinate chicken with 15ml soy sauce, ginger, garlic (30 mins)
2. Heat wok until smoking, add oil
3. Stir fry chicken until golden (4-5 mins), remove
4. Stir fry vegetables (3-4 mins)
5. Return chicken, add sauce, cook 2 mins
6. Garnish and serve with rice

Serves 4

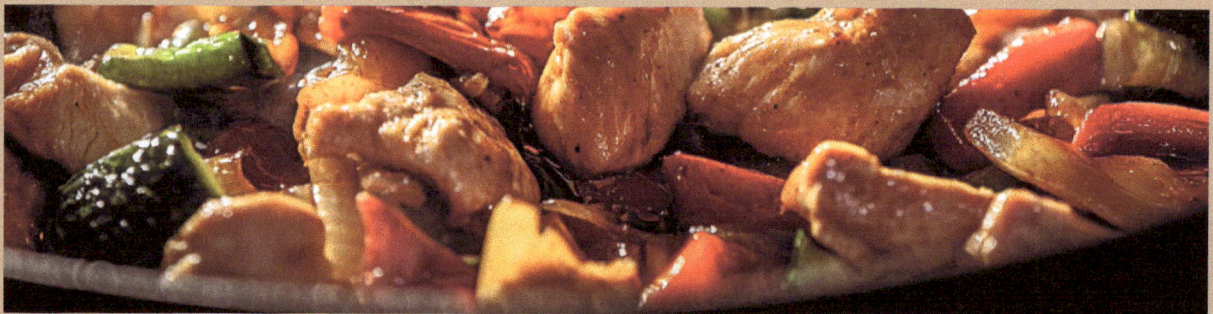

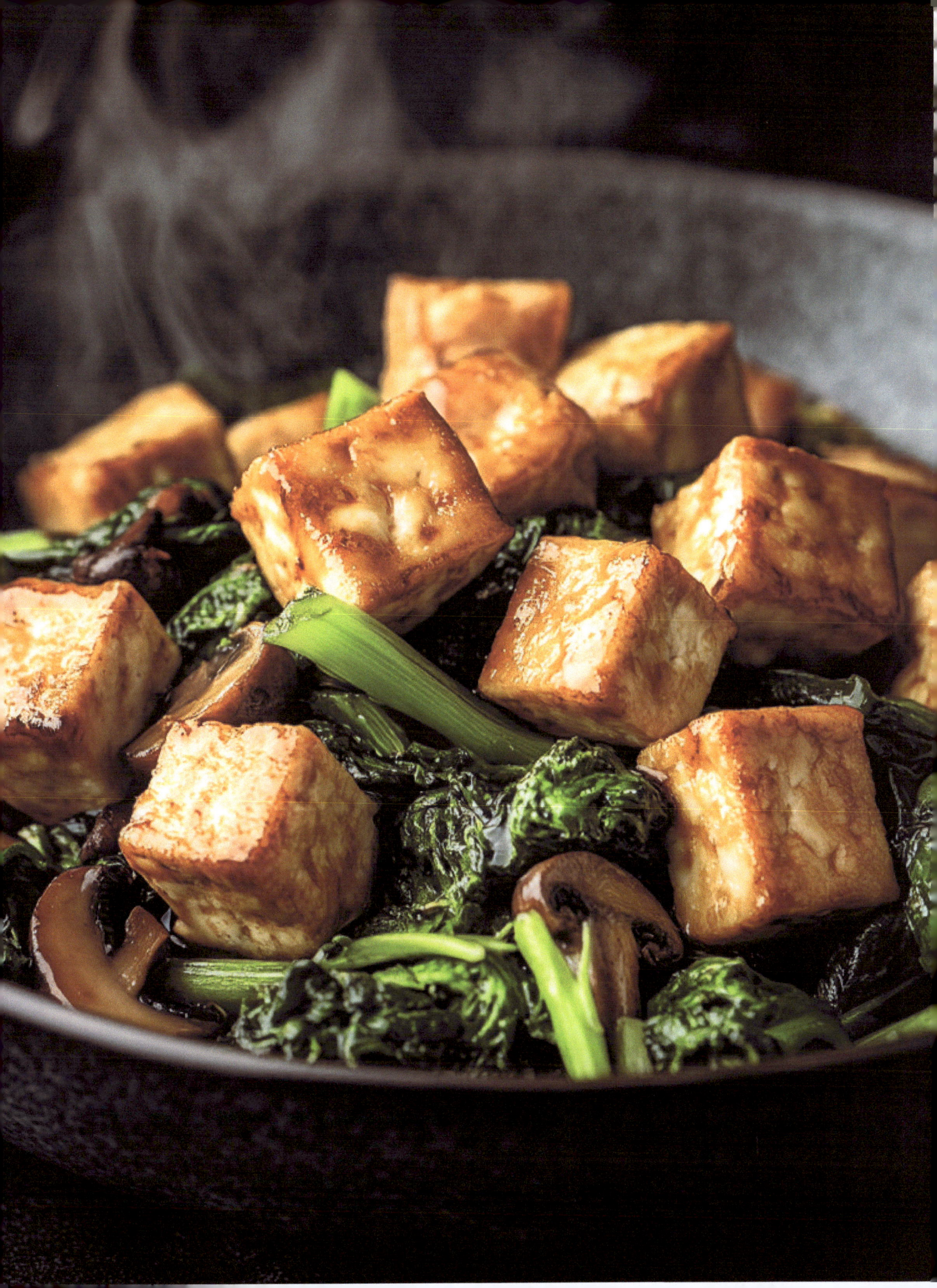

Spicy Tofu & Mushroom Stir Fry:

INGREDIENTS

400g firm tofu, pressed and cubed
250g mushrooms, sliced
2 cups snap peas
1 cup edamame
30ml chili garlic sauce

Sauce: 30ml tamari, 15ml rice vinegar, 5ml sesame oil

Garnish: crushed peanuts

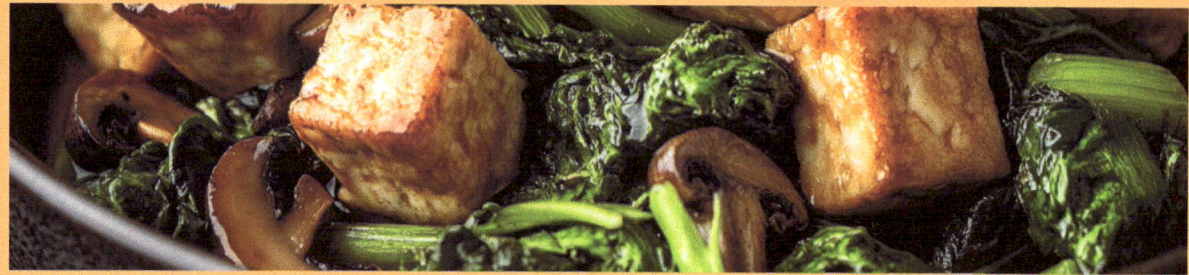

METHOD

1. Press tofu between paper towels (30 mins)
2. Heat wok until smoking, add oil
3. Fry tofu until golden (5-6 mins), remove
4. Stir fry mushrooms (3 mins)
5. Add remaining vegetables (2-3 mins)
6. Return tofu, add sauce and chili garlic sauce
7. Cook 2 mins, garnish with peanuts

Serves 4

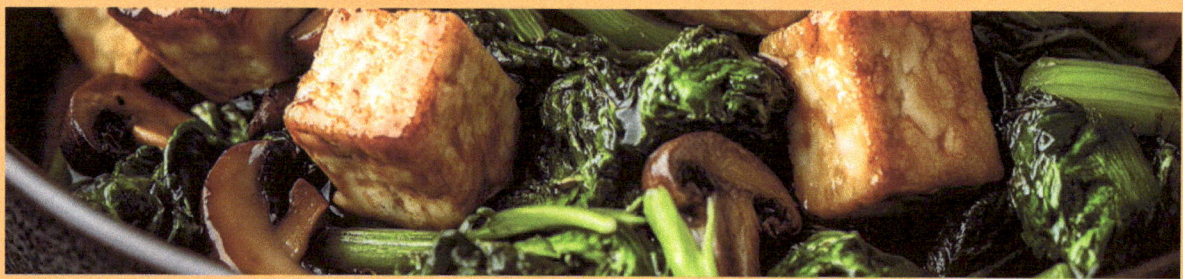

From Couch to Karate
My Return to Martial Arts
by Peter Thompson

I never thought I'd be writing this story. At 46, staring at blood pressure readings that made my doctor wince and carrying an extra 15 kilos, I was forced to confront a harsh reality. My dad's heart attack wasn't just a tragedy – it was a warning.

Sitting in my doctor's office, those words hit hard: "Pete, you're heading down the same path as your father." The memory of Dad's funeral was still fresh. I'd spent weeks afterwards looking at old photos, including ones from my teenage karate days. I barely recognised that fit, confident kid in the white gi.

Walking into the local dojo nearly broke me. The familiar smell of sweat and polish brought back memories, but my reflection in the mirror told a different story. Sensei Mike, though, he was different from what I expected. No drill sergeant attitude, just genuine understanding.

"Listen, mate," he said, noticing my hesitation, "everyone here started somewhere. Let's just focus on getting you moving again."

Those first few weeks were humbling. Simple things like basic stances left me gasping. My knees cracked during squats, and my kicks wouldn't have scared a paper bag. But Sensei Mike had a plan.

We started with fundamentals:
- 15 minutes of gentle stretching
- Basic punching techniques
- Simple kata movements
- Core strengthening exercises

The hardest part? Accepting that I couldn't do what I did at 16. "Your body's got different memories now," Sensei Mike explained. "We need to create new ones."

Changing Habits

It wasn't just about training. I had to look at everything:
- Swapped my morning pie for overnight oats
- Started walking during lunch breaks
- Cut back on beers (mostly)
- Actually listened to my body when it needed rest

Three months in, something unexpected happened. My 15-year-old son Jack started showing interest. "Dad, can I come to class?" Those words changed everything. Suddenly, I wasn't just fighting for my health – I was setting an example.

We cleared out the garage, laid down some mats. Now we practice together most nights. Even my daughter joins in sometimes, though she reckons we look like uncoordinated pandas.

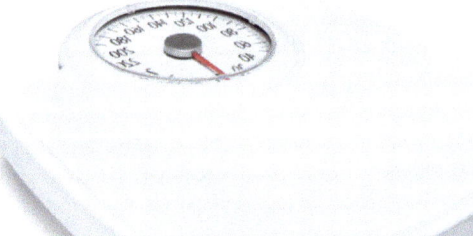

Nine months later, I'm 12 kilos lighter. My blood pressure's normal, and I've just earned my green belt. But the real changes aren't physical. I sleep better. I have more energy. Most importantly, I'm showing my kids that it's never too late to turn things around.

Lessons Learned

For anyone thinking about returning to martial arts:
- Find a sensei who understands older beginners
- Accept your current limitations
- Document your progress (those small wins matter)
- Keep your ego in check
- Get your family involved - somehow
- Remember why you started

Some days still hurt. My roundhouse kicks won't win any beauty contests, and I still modify certain exercises. But that's okay. This journey isn't about becoming a champion – it's about becoming healthier, stronger, and being around longer for my family.

Dad would've been proud. Not of the belts or the techniques, but of the decision to change. Sometimes the bravest thing we can do is admit we need to start over.

Looking forward I've got new goals now. Nothing fancy – just steady improvement. My next challenge is a local tournament in the veterans' division. Not to win, mind you, just to prove to myself that I can.

If you're reading this, sitting on the fence about starting again, just take that first step. The hardest belt to earn isn't black – it's the one that gets you through the door.

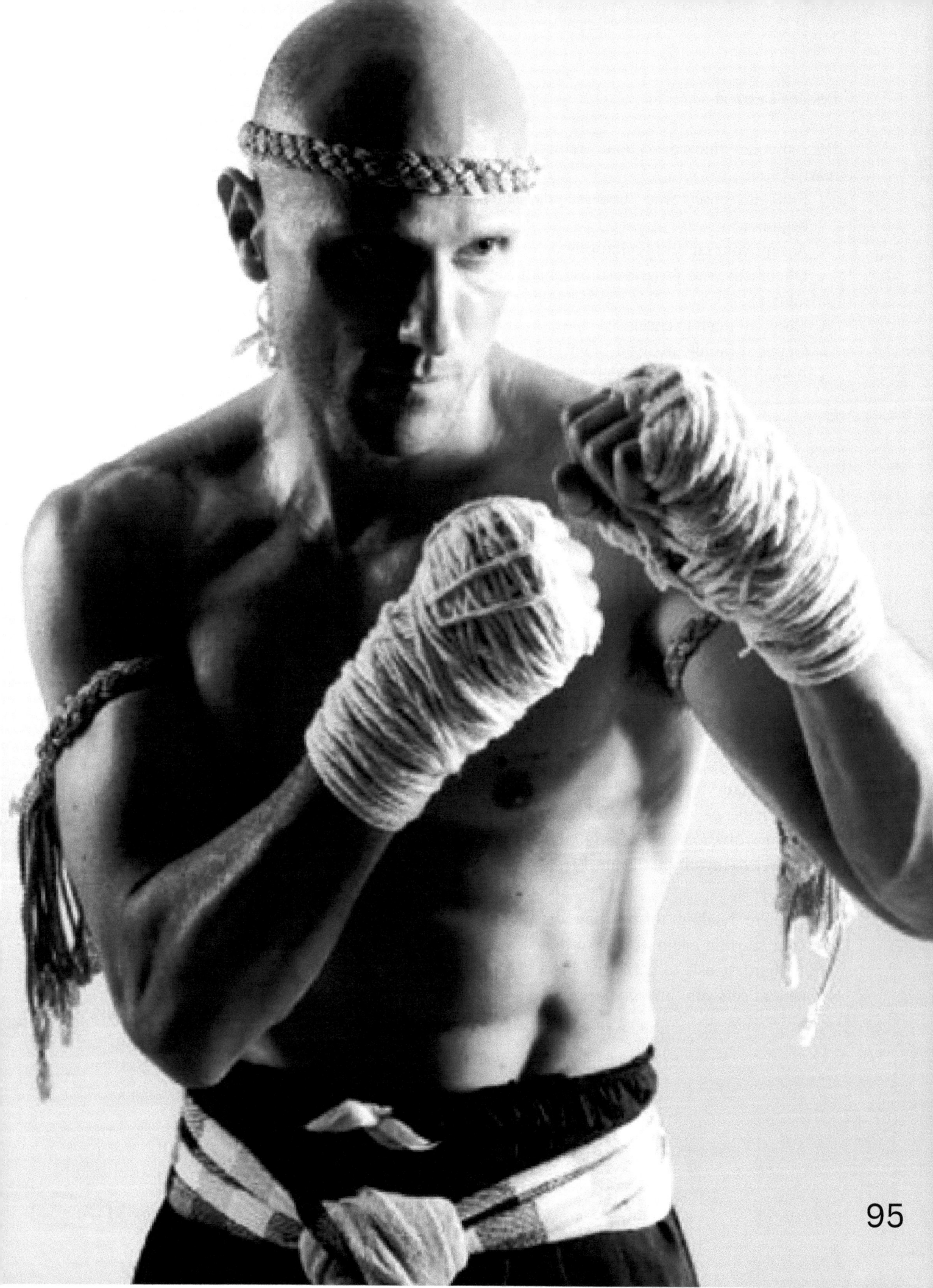

IMBA

The International Muay Boran Academy

The International Muay Boran Academy (IMBA) is the first international school devoted to the development of traditional Thai unarmed fighting disciplines (since 1993). IMBA has been created thanks to the dedication of one of the most renowned worldwide exponents of Muay Thai, the Italian Master Marco De Cesaris, founder and technical director of IMBA.

In the last few years, the International Muay Boran Academy has successfully created a global network of highly qualified Muay Thai Boran instructors in Europe, Latin America and Oceania. Over the past 20 years, the International Academy founded by Master Marco De Cesaris, has concentrated all its efforts on the re-organisation and dissemination of Thailand's forgotten unarmed combat techniques. The conventional name chosen to denote this ancient martial discipline was Muay Thai Boran; a set of forgotten techniques designed over the centuries by the Kingdom of Siam's masters.

> Muay Thai Boran as it is practised in all IMBA Branches worldwide is fully combat oriented: its main goal is making men and women ready for all-out fighting. For this reason, all IMBA members are welcome to take part in technical seminars held regularly; advanced seminars are devoted to the deeper understandings of ancient fighting techniques and strategies (i.e., Mae Mai-Look Mai Muay Thai, Chern Muay, Kon Muay Kae) and their combative applications with a special attention on their use in self-defence.

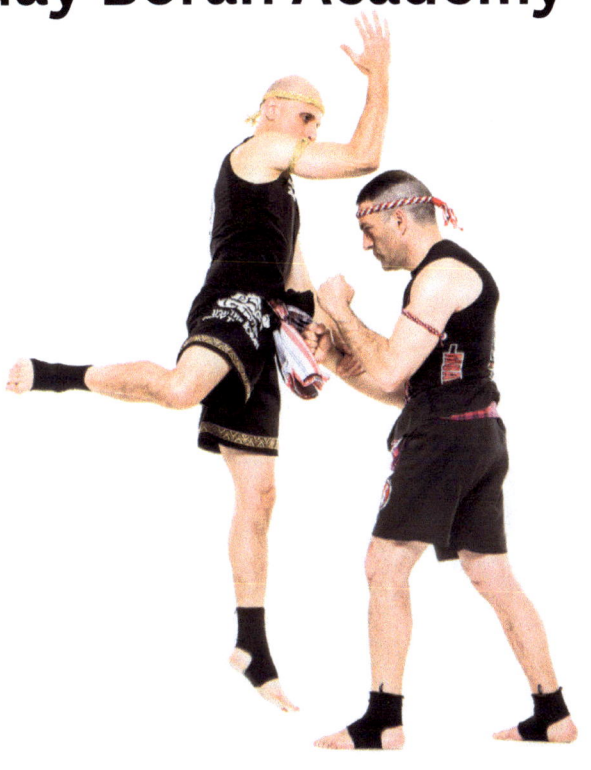

Open courses for instructors are frequently staged both locally and internationally, and Khan grading sessions for students and instructors are held regularly. IMBA Muay Boran is a complete fighting art that combines the ring fighting science of Muay Thai with the martial applications of ancient Siamese unarmed combat techniques. In encouraging the two different aspects of the art to coexist, IMBA Muay Boran successfully bridges the gap between modern combat sports and traditional martial arts.

Thanks to the effort of all IMBA members worldwide, traditional Muay has finally become a true world heritage, as advocated by the Thai masters of old time.

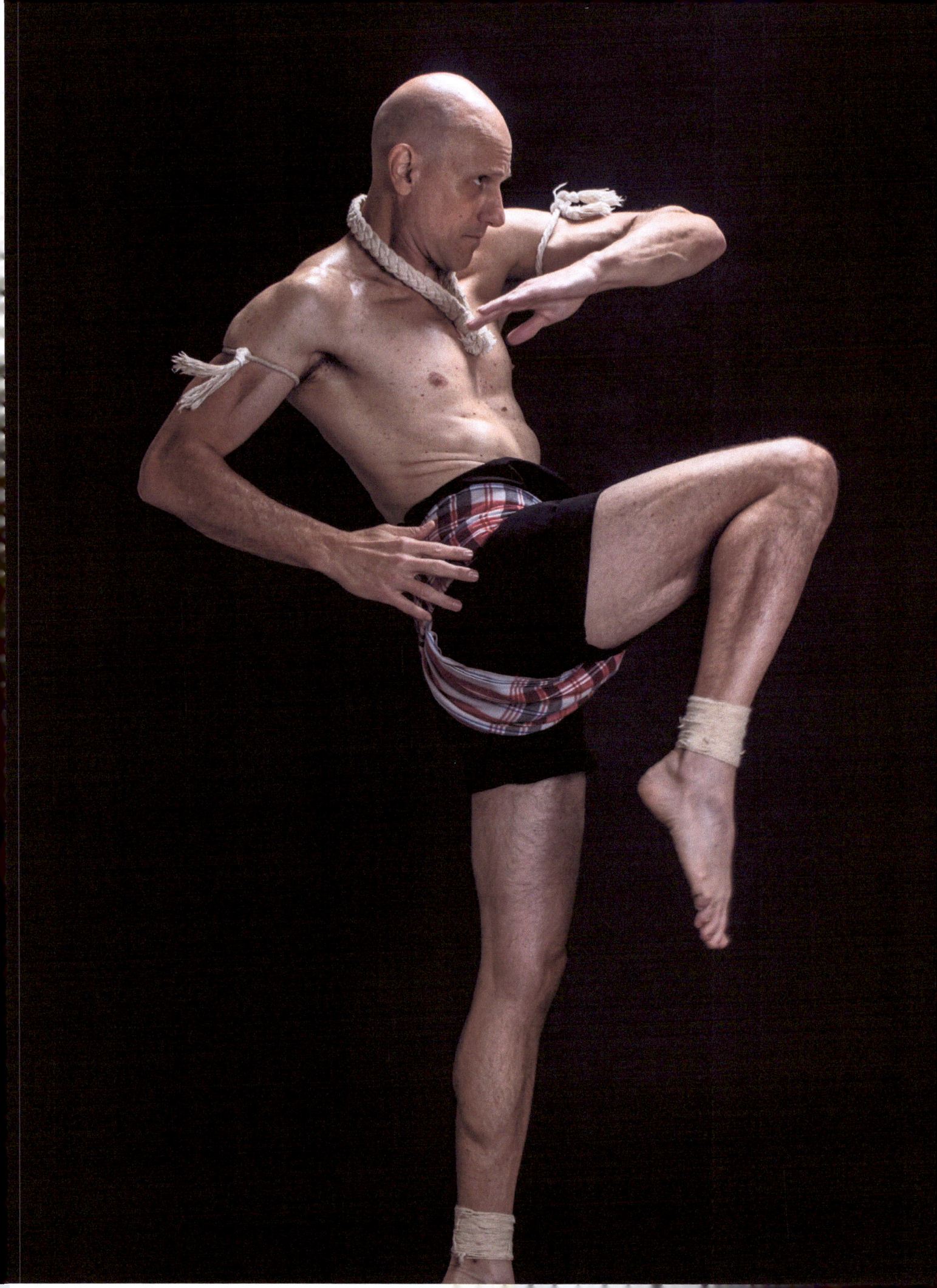

Combat Muay Boran (the most combative interpretation of the original unarmed Thai martial arts' fighting skills), IMBA Lert Rit (a Siamese military Close Combat style adapted to civilian use) and IMBA Muay Pram (the present-day version of classical Thai Grappling) represent the three technical pillars of IMBA Muay Boran, the modern and scientific version of original Muay Thai Boran, developed since 2005.

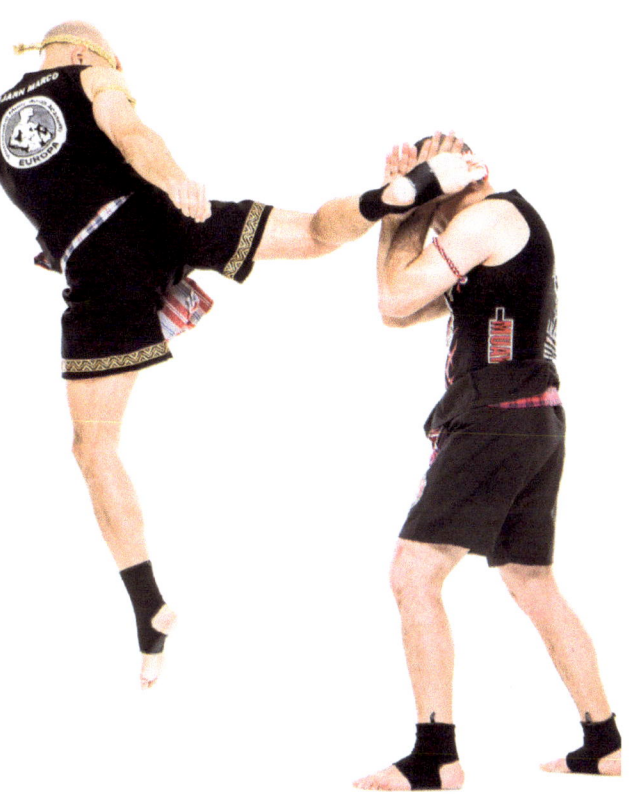

Master Marco has been a Muay Thai practitioner since 1978 and has been certified as a teacher of Muay by the Ministry of Education of Thailand (in 1991). During his career, he was an athlete, coach of professional Thai boxers, judge / referee, promoter and founder of the first Italian Muay Thai Federation. In the year 2007, he was awarded the Gold Medal in the World Muay Boran Championships, solo Technical Forms competition, held at Bangkok National Stadium. In 2012, he was awarded the 15th Khan of Muay Thai Boran (and the title of Bramarjarn or Grand Master of the Art) and the Gold Mongkon by the Governor of Ayutthaya Province, Thailand.

IMBA is in its novice stages of introducing its curriculum to Australia. Classes have commenced in Perth and are looking to extend to all states.

For further information on classes please contact:
Australian Representative: Kru Maria Quaglia at imbaaust@gmail.com.au .
Website: www.muaythai.it
YouTube: https://youtube.com/@MuaythaiIt?si=cOeBshBP9AzuBQwo

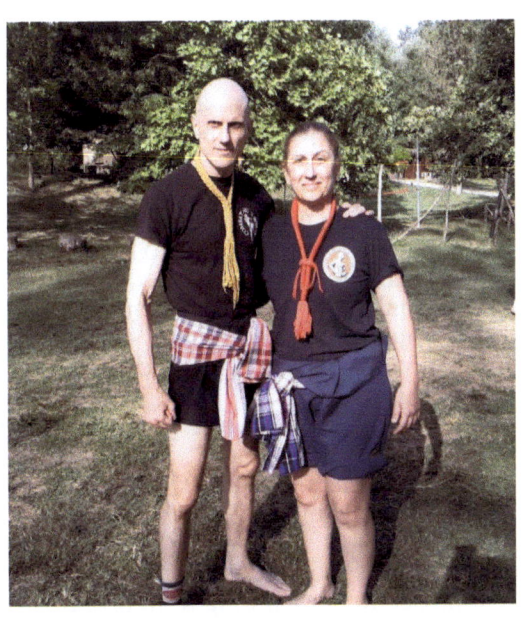

Kru Maria Quaglia with Master Marco

Ask the Dojo Doctor

I'm a beginner in MMA, and I often experience pain in my wrists during training. What can I do to prevent this?

Wrist pain is a common issue for beginners in martial arts. To prevent this, make sure you're using proper technique when punching or blocking. Keep your wrist straight and aligned with your forearm. You can also perform wrist strengthening exercises, such as wrist curls and reverse wrist curls, to build strength and stability.

Additionally, consider using wrist wraps or supports during training to provide extra protection and support. If the pain persists or worsens, consult with your instructor or a medical professional.

I've been training in martial arts for a while, but I feel like I've hit a plateau in my progress. How can I continue to improve?

Plateaus are a normal part of any martial arts journey. To break through and continue improving, try the following:

1. Set specific goals: identify areas where you want to improve and set measurable goals to work towards.
2. Vary your training: incorporate different drills, techniques, and training methods to challenge your body and mind in new ways.
3. Cross-train: explore other martial arts styles or complementary practices like yoga or weightlifting to develop a well-rounded skill set.
4. Analyze your performance: record yourself during training or sparring and review the footage to identify areas for improvement.
5. Seek feedback: ask your instructor or training partners for constructive criticism and advice on how to refine your technique.

Remember, consistent practice and a growth mindset are key to long-term progress

After a considerable break I have returned to training at a local dojo. I was previously a black belt and the new style allow me to wear my black belt to class which I thought was a good thing because I feel I am too old to go back to being a white belt. The trouble is this new style is way more complex than my previous style and I am really feeling out of place. What can I do to catch up without becoming a liability in every class I attend?

Returning to martial arts after a break can be challenging, especially when joining a new style that is more complex than your previous one. Here are some tips to help you catch up and avoid feeling like a liability in class:

1. Discuss your situation with your instructor, letting them know about your previous experience and your desire to catch up. They may be able to provide you with additional guidance, resources, or private lessons to help you bridge the gap.
2. Even though you're wearing a black belt, don't hesitate to spend extra time practicing the fundamental techniques of the new style. Mastering the basics will provide a solid foundation for learning more advanced techniques.
3. After each class, write down the techniques, drills, and concepts you learned. Review your notes between classes to reinforce your understanding and identify areas where you need more practice.
4. Dedicate time to practicing techniques and forms on your own. This will allow you to progress at your own pace and build muscle memory.
5. Don't be afraid to ask your instructor or advanced students for clarification or advice when you're unsure about a technique or concept. Most martial artists are happy to help others learn and grow.
6. Learning a new style takes time, so don't be too hard on yourself if you feel like you're not progressing as quickly as you'd like. Celebrate your small victories and improvements along the way.

Everyone in class is there to learn and grow, regardless of rank. By consistently putting in the effort and maintaining a positive attitude, you'll soon find yourself catching up and contributing to the dojo's community.

Write for Us

We want your authentic story, your journey and the reason WHY you love what you do. Below is a list of suggested topics. It is not exhaustive, so if you have an idea that we haven't come up with yet, drop us a line: training tips; technique workshops; style origins;kids in ma; training fuel; style anatomy; family pages; instructor profile; keeping it real; and more...

We are a quarterly magazine that celebrates and inspires a broad community of Martial Artists across the country. Our goal is to support all MA practitioners. Both instructors and students are encouraged to share their personal experiences, triumphs, and challenges within the style they love.

We feature interviews, rants, research, photography, projects and editorials that are respectful to all styles and are keeping in line with our magazine's inclusive philosophy.

Just as no two styles of Martial Arts are alike, our writers should have their own unique voice and tell their story from their own perspective. We encourage you to speak your truth.

Don't worry if you feel that your writing is not up to scratch, just tell us your story, your tip or your instruction the best way you can and our in-house editor will do the rest.

Email your submissions to info@martialartsmagazineaustralia.com (text in .doc) and (photos in JPEG).

Printed by Libri Plureos GmbH in Hamburg, Germany